"The Object Lessons series achieves something very close to magic: the books take ordinary—even banal—objects and animate them with a rich history of invention, political struggle, science, and popular mythology. Filled with fascinating details and conveyed in sharp, accessible prose, the books make the everyday world come to life. Be warned: once you've read a few of these, you'll start walking around your house, picking up random objects, and musing aloud: 'I wonder what the story is behind this thing?'"

Steven Johnson, author of *Where Good Ideas Come From* and *How We Got to Now*

"Object Lessons describes themselves as 'short, beautiful books,' and to that, I'll say, amen. . . . If you read enough Object Lessons books, you'll fill your head with plenty of trivia to amaze and annoy your friends and loved ones—caution recommended on pontificating on the objects surrounding you. More importantly, though . . . they inspire us to take a second look at parts of the everyday that we've taken for granted. These are not so much lessons about the objects themselves, but opportunities for self-reflection and storytelling. They remind us that we are surrounded by a wondrous world, as long as we care to look."

John Warner, *The Chicago Tribune*

T0266576

"Besides being beautiful little hand-sized objects themselves, showcasing exceptional writing, the wonder of these books is that they exist at all . . . Uniformly excellent, engaging, thought-provoking, and informative."

Jennifer Bort Yacovissi, *Washington Independent Review of Books*

". . . edifying and entertaining . . . perfect for slipping in a pocket and pulling out when life is on hold."

Sarah Murdoch, *Toronto Star*

"For my money, Object Lessons is the most consistently interesting nonfiction book series in America."

PopMatters

"Though short, at roughly 25,000 words apiece, these books are anything but slight."

Marina Benjamin, *New Statesman*

"[W]itty, thought-provoking, and poetic . . . These little books are a page-flipper's dream."

John Timpane, *The Philadelphia Inquirer*

The joy of the series, of reading *Remote Control*, *Golf Ball*, *Driver's License*, *Drone*, *Silence*, *Glass*, *Refrigerator*, *Hotel*, and *Waste* (more titles are listed as forthcoming) in quick succession, lies in encountering the various turns through which each of their authors has been put by his or her object. As for Benjamin, so for the authors of the series, the object predominates, sits squarely center stage, directs the action. The object decides the genre, the chronology, and the limits of the study. Accordingly, the author has to take her cue from the *thing* she chose or that chose her. The result is a wonderfully uneven series of books, each one a *thing* unto itself."

Julian Yates, *Los Angeles Review of Books*

The Object Lessons series has a beautifully simple premise. Each book or essay centers on a specific object. This can be mundane or unexpected, humorous or politically timely. Whatever the subject, these descriptions reveal the rich worlds hidden under the surface of things."

Christine Ro, *Book Riot*

. . . a sensibility somewhere between Roland Barthes and Wes Anderson."

Simon Reynolds, author of *Retromania: Pop Culture's Addiction to Its Own Past*

My favourite series of short pop culture books"

Zoomer magazine

OBJECTLESSONS

A book series about the hidden lives of ordinary things.

Series Editors:

Ian Bogost and Christopher Schaberg

In association with

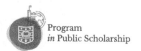

BOOKS IN THE SERIES

X-ray

NICOLE LOBDELL

BLOOMSBURY ACADEMIC
NEW YORK · LONDON · OXFORD · NEW DELHI · SYDNEY

BLOOMSBURY ACADEMIC
Bloomsbury Publishing Inc
1385 Broadway, New York, NY 10018, USA
50 Bedford Square, London, WC1B 3DP, UK
29 Earlsfort Terrace, Dublin 2, Ireland

BLOOMSBURY, BLOOMSBURY ACADEMIC and the Diana logo are trademarks of Bloomsbury
Publishing Plc

First published in the United States of America 2024

Copyright © Nicole Lobdell, 2024

Cover design: Alice Marwick

For legal purposes the List of Figures on p. xii constitute an extension of this copyright page.

All rights reserved. No part of this publication may be reproduced or transmitted in any form or by
any means, electronic or mechanical, including photocopying, recording, or any information
storage or retrieval system, without prior permission in writing from the publishers.

Bloomsbury Publishing Inc does not have any control over, or responsibility for, any third-party
websites referred to or in this book. All internet addresses given in this book were correct at the
time of going to press. The author and publisher regret any inconvenience caused if addresses
have changed or sites have ceased to exist, but can accept no responsibility for any such changes.

Whilst every effort has been made to locate copyright holders the publishers would be grateful to
hear from any person(s) not here acknowledged.

Library of Congress Cataloging-in-Publication Data

Names: Lobdell, Nicole, author.
Title: X-ray / Nicole Lobdell.
Description: New York: Bloomsbury Academic, 2024. | Series: Object lessons |
Includes bibliographical references and index.
Identifiers: LCCN 2023055222 (print) | LCCN 2023055223 (ebook) | ISBN 9781501386701
(paperback) | ISBN 9781501386718 (ebook) | ISBN 9781501386725 (pdf)
Subjects: LCSH: X-rays. | X-rays–Social aspects. | X-rays–History. | X-rays–Therapeutic use.
Classification: LCC QC481 .L63 2024 (print) | LCC QC481 (ebook) |
DDC 616.07/572–dc23/eng/20240129
LC record available at https://lccn.loc.gov/2023055222
LC ebook record available at https://lccn.loc.gov/2023055223

ISBN: PB: 978-1-5013-8670-1
ePDF: 978-1-5013-8672-5
eBook: 978-1-5013-867-1-8

Series: Object Lessons

Typeset by Deanta Global Publishing Services, Chennai, India
Printed and bound in Great Britain.

To find out more about our authors and books visit www.bloomsbury.com and sign up
for our newsletters.

For those who see through me:
Harry, Lisa, Deepa, Robert, Ryan, and Betsy

CONTENTS

FIGURES

1 DISCOVERY

"X is crossed swords, a battle: who will win? We do not know, so the mystics made it the sign of destiny and the algebraists the sign of the unknown"

— VICTOR HUGO

On November 8, 1895, while experimenting with passing cathode rays (streams of electrons) through a Crookes tube (a glass tube containing a partial vacuum and a positive electrode on one end and a negative electrode at the other end), German physicist Wilhelm Conrad Roentgen observed a fluorescent screen across the room began to glow. With further experimentation, he discovered that objects placed between the tube and the fluorescent screen created shadow-like images on the screen behind them. He began placing larger and more diverse objects in the pathway: a letter in a sealed envelope, a 1000-page book, a set of weights in a wooden box, and his own hunting rifle. Even when he covered the tube so that it emitted no visible light, the invisible rays

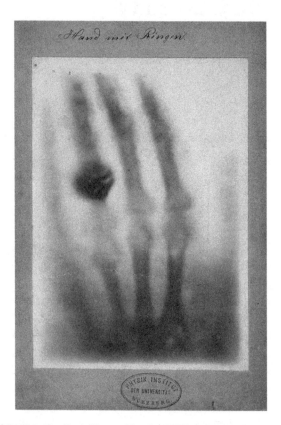

FIGURE 1 *Hand mit Ringen* (Hand with Ring): a print of one of the first X-rays by Wilhelm Roentgen (1845–1923) of the left hand of his wife Anna Bertha. Credit: Wellcome Collection, London. Wellcome Images. Creative Commons Attribution 4.0 International.

continued to pass through objects. For nearly two months, Roentgen secretly devoted himself to experimenting with these new rays. He told no one of his discovery, not even his wife Anna Bertha, who brought him meals in his lab when he forgot to eat. Then, on December 22, 1895, six weeks after his initial experiment, Roentgen asked his wife to place her hand in the pathway. She did. After fifteen minutes of exposure, the image of a skeletal hand appeared on the screen. Upon seeing it, she exclaimed: "I have seen my death!" Despite Anna's initial fears and misgivings, Roentgen shared the image with the world, publishing it along with his report "On a New Kind of Rays" on January 1, 1896. Until that day, the power to see into the hearts of men had belonged solely to the gods. Now, it belonged to men.

X-rays are many things. They are invisible beams of light, haunting pictures, superpowers, and metaphors. As light, X-rays exist on a part of the electromagnetic spectrum invisible to the human eye, but they are all around us. To paraphrase Timothy Morton: we don't see them—they see us. X-rays are photographs of the body moving through time; palimpsests of the past, present, and future. X-rays are paradoxes, reproducing themselves as they turn the world inside out. In 1896, the X-ray was a portal, a port hole, offering a view of the hidden world inside. In an era of technological innovation that sought to explore the world outside (railways, electric lights, telegrams), the X-ray looked inward. And after Roentgen published his findings, no one was safe from the X-ray's gaze.

News of Roentgen's discovery spread like lightning, and because Roentgen had designed his machine with easily obtainable parts—a Crookes vacuum tube and an electrical current—amateur scientists and hobbyists could DIY their very own X-ray machines—and they did! Affluent families even installed X-ray machines in their homes, using them as entertainment for evening parties, while innovators and inventors, like Edison, immediately set to work improving upon Roentgen's design. Within two years, there were dozens of books, hundreds of articles, and at least thirty different types of X-ray bulbs that could see farther and penetrate deeper. The existence of invisible X-ray light on the electromagnetic spectrum proved the limitations of human eyesight, but X-rays were also the obvious tools for overcoming it. By harnessing the power of X-rays, Roentgen not only opened a portal to a new world—he gave the world new eyes with which to see it.

In publishing his discovery, Roentgen made two important decisions. The first was the choice of name. What's in a name? Everything. If friends of Roentgen had had their way, we would call them "Roentgen Rays." A humble man, Roentgen deferred. In *La Géométrie* (1637), Rene Descartes uses "X" as a mathematical substitute for an unknown variable. A true scientist, Roentgen named them X-rays because he did not know what the rays were made of. They were a true unknown—an "X." Roentgen put his scientific principles first and gave X-rays the name that most accurately reflected their nature. What Roentgen couldn't know at the time was the power of his branding.

X is a powerful letter. We love it for its mystery and its promise of something undefined but extraordinary. From *X-Men* and *X-Files* to Malcom X and Generation X, X signifies the unknown, the rebel, the off-limits, and the taboo. Put an X before a word and it denotes mystery—the X factor. Put it after a word or a name and it suggests rebellion, resistance, and rebirth. After he came out as a gay music artist, singer Lil Nas renamed himself Lil Nas X.

The poet Joshua Bennett praises X for its breadth, seeing in it a symbol of power and possibility for himself and the Black community:

As you are both Malcolm's
shadow & the black unknown
he died defending, I praise

your untold potential, the possible
worlds you hold within your body's
bladed frame. I love how you stand

in exultation, arms raised
[...]

—"X" by Joshua Bennett[1]

As a symbol, X warns of danger, from railroad crossing signs and chemical hazard signs, to the skull and crossbones. It has the power to halt us in our tracks. Or, X marks the spot, compelling us onward to adventure, to discover what lies beneath. X entices—XOXO, X-rated, XXX—as well as deletes—to cross out, to ex out a wrong answer. X symbolizes life—X and Y chromosomes—and death, x_x. With X, we can multiple (2 x 2) and measure (2' x 2'), cross stitch and collaborate: Jane x Bob, you x me. With X, we make our mark. With X-rays, Roentgen made his.

After naming his discovery X-rays, the second most important decision Roentgen made was in publishing the X-ray image of Anna Bertha's hand. It is this decision that changed the world. By choosing an X-ray of a human hand as the very first X-ray the world saw, Roentgen demonstrated the immediate medical implications of X-ray technology, as he had hoped.

Within days of Roentgen's publication, X-rays of human hands began appearing by the dozens in publications around the world. From Berlin to Baltimore, scientists as well as amateurs followed Roentgen's instructions, built their own X-ray devices, and began X-raying their hands. If Instagram had been around, it would have been full of skeletal hands.

Within weeks of publication, X-rays were in service in hospitals for the sick and on battlefields for the injured. In January 1896, less than a month after Roentgen's publication, Michael I. Pupin, a Columbia University X-ray and electrical innovator (whose induction coil design made long-distance phone calls a reality), took a historic X-ray photograph of a man's left hand with over forty shotgun pellets lodged in it from a hunting accident. Like other early X-ray innovators,

Pupin had experimented with and modified Roentgen's X-ray machine designs, devising a method for producing X-ray images within minutes rather than hours. When the injured man was brought to his laboratory, Pupin quickly produced the X-ray, revealing the extent of the man's injuries and demonstrating one of the first applications of a near-instant X-ray imagining in a medical emergency. Today, X-ray imagining in medical emergencies seems commonplace, banal even, but in January 1896, it was the cutting edge of medical technology.

The first recorded usage of X-ray machines in service on the battlefield was by the British army in 1897 outside Cairo, where the British field hospital installed an X-ray machine. In 1898, when war with Spain broke out, the US Army outfitted three hospital ships with X-ray machines, which the US Army Medical Department later claimed had "done away with the necessity for exploration of wounds by probes [and] . . . obviated the dangers of infection and additional [traumas]."[2] The most famous instances of X-rays on battlefields were Marie Curie's X-ray vans of the First World War. Winner of the Nobel Prize for Physics in 1903 and for Chemistry in 1911, Curie designed and outfitted vans with mobile X-ray machines. They became known as "Little Curies." In addition to raising money and recruiting and training 150 women to drive and operate the X-ray machines, Curie herself drove one on the front lines of battle. It's impossible to estimate how many lives were saved because of prompt medical imagining and Curie's foresight.

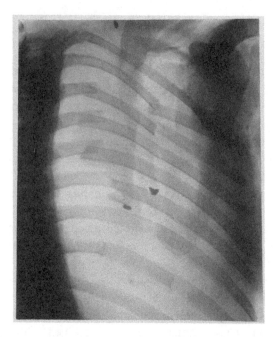

FIGURE 2 Chest X-ray of Corporal Douglas Herbert Phillips, died November 24, 1915. "X-rays of First World War Wounds," Professor Thomas Renton Elliott Collection. Credit: Wellcome Collection, London.

X-rays themselves, however, are not curative, and the medical archives produced during the First World War are full of X-rays from soldiers who did not survive their injuries. In a box of X-rays from the First World War at the Wellcome Collection Medical Museum and Library in London, I came across the chest X-ray of a soldier named Phillips who served during the First World War in the 7th Northamptons. According to the medical notes that accompanied it, on November 16, 1915, Phillips suffered a "tangential shell wound of back of chest splitting left scapula from above downwards."[3] The impact left Phillips with five broken ribs, a broken scapula, and several other fractures. The medical notes indicate infection set in: "haemo-pneumothorax of 50 ozs. infected with streptococci and staphylococci."[4] In other words, Phillips had fifty ounces of blood (haemo) and air (pneumo) in the space between the linings of his lungs (the pleural cavity), which allowed pneumonia (streptococci) and infection (staphylococci) to take hold. In 1915, the antibiotics needed to treat pneumonia and infection did not yet exist. Penicillin, for example, would not be available until 1928. With these injuries, Phillips would have fought for every breath, and every breath would have been agony. While the X-ray could show medical staff the severity of Phillips's injuries, it could do little else but confirm what they already knew—Phillips would not survive. Eight days later, as the X-ray had divined, Phillips succumbed to his injuries. His official cause of death was listed as pneumonia and pericarditis, inflammation of the sack around the heart. Holding Phillips's chest X-ray in my hands as I read the medical notes and comprehended what they meant, I found myself overwhelmed. The gray archival box containing dozens of similar X-rays took on the appearance of a mass grave.

X-rays are deeply intimate, but they also run the risk of being impersonal. These X-rays of life-ending injuries offered no first names, a double erasure. Before I returned Phillips's X-ray, the image of his death that I held in my hands, I wanted to restore his identity. I found him listed among the casualties of the First World War. Phillips was Corporal Douglas Herbert Phillips, the 24-year-old son of Herbert and Elizabeth Phillips of Abington Park Crescent, Northampton. Buried in the Boulogne Eastern Cemetery in the Pas de Calais region of France, someone, his parents perhaps, chose John 15:13 as his epitaph: "Greater love hath no man than this, that a man lay down his life for his friends."

X-rays help people make sense of death. Perhaps it's no surprise then that within weeks of Roentgen's discovery, the first X-rays of ancient death were developed and published by German physicist Walter Koenig. In March 1896, Koenig X-rayed the mummified remains of an ancient Egyptian child at the Senckenberg Museum of Natural History in Germany. The images allowed Koenig and others to identify previously unknown anatomical features of the child, including clues as to the child's sex (male) and age (four to five years old, based on the teeth). With this, the field of paleoradiology was born.

X-rays gave researchers and scientists the chance to study ancient remains and artifacts without unwrapping or irrevocably damaging them. In 1896, X-ray images of mummified remains revealed to researchers ancient secrets, artifacts hidden beneath wrappings, burial rites, and signs of disease and injury. In 1903, the first ancient Egyptian royal mummy X-rayed was Thutmose IV, the eighth pharaoh of the 18th dynasty who reigned in the 14th century BCE. The images established the royal's approximate age at the time of his death. X-rays also allowed historians to date ancient Egyptian remains more accurately based on the positioning of the arms, which were often not visible under the wrappings. The arm placement, whether at the sides, high across the chest, or low across the chest, is indicative of the dynasty to which the person belonged as burial practices changed with time. Previously, these details were often unknown or only loosely guessed at. Now with good X-ray images, historians and researchers could make important discoveries that offered new understandings of a historic civilization.

Bad X-rays, however, could lead to wrong conclusions. The most famous of these involves the supposed murder of King Tutankhamen, the great-grandson of Thutmose IV, who ascended the Egyptian throne at eight years old and died when he was nineteen. In 1967, a team from the University of Michigan partnered with Alexandria University in Egypt to X-ray the royal mummy collection in the Egyptian Museum in Cairo for a groundbreaking study titled *An X-ray Atlas of Royal Mummies* (1980). There were problems from the beginning. The X-ray equipment was poor, and the team was not allowed to X-ray the remains outside their leaded glass cases. What's the one thing that can stop X-rays? Lead. Taking X-rays through leaded glass creates image distortion, but researchers did not account for the distortion in their analysis. When studying the

X-rays of Tutankhamen, researchers saw bone fragments in the skull and interpreted them—wrongly, many would argue—as signs of blunt-force trauma. Based on these interpretations, historians speculated that Tutankhamen was murdered. This theory quickly became the leading theory of his death for over 35 years. Researchers never considered that the bone fragments might be from the deterioration of the skull caused when Tutankhamen's tomb was discovered and disturbed in 1922 by Howard Carter. In 2006 and with the use of advanced CT imagining, it was revealed that infection from a broken femur combined with multiple weaknesses, or possibly disease, were most likely the cause of the boy-king's death. Nevertheless, rumors of his murder persist.

Using X-rays as evidence of a crime is not new. *Smith v. Grant*, the first court case dependent on the use of X-rays as evidence, was heard in April 1896, just six months after Roentgen's discovery. In *Smith v. Grant*, James Smith, a young man injured in a fall from a ladder, sued Dr. William West Grant, the surgeon who examined Smith's injuries and, despite having fractured a femur in the fall, advised Smith to exercise. Smith sued Grant for medical malpractice because Grant failed to diagnose him correctly and prescribed him treatment that resulted in further injury. Smith's lawyer introduced the X-ray images, which he had taken especially for the lawsuit, as evidence of Grant's negligence. It worked. Convinced by the X-ray evidence of Smith's injuries, the judged ruled in Smith's favor.

In 1896, most people had very little understanding of what X-rays were or how X-rays worked. Nevertheless, just like today, legal systems had to account for the new technology, sometimes in unpredictable ways. In January 1896, after reading about X-rays in the newspaper, one man sent his opera glasses to Thomas Edison at his laboratory in West Orange, New Jersey, with the request that Edison "fit them with the 'X-rays' and return them."[5] Presumably, it was this report that caused Assemblyman Charles A. Reed of Somerset County, New Jersey in February 1896 to introduce a bill "prohibiting the use of X-rays in opera glasses in theaters."[6]

Through X-rays, many people saw a world of awesome possibilities. The temperance movement hoped X-rays would prove the harmful effects of alcohol on the body's internal organs, while the spiritualist movement believed X-rays would prove the existence of the soul. One New York newspaper earnestly reported "that at the College of Physicians and Surgeons the roentgen rays were used to reflect anatomic diagrams directly into the brains of the students," suggesting this method would teach students to retain the information faster and more accurately.[7] Edison was falsely rumored to have cured blindness with X-rays, a rumor that would persist for years. Others imagined ways that X-rays might improve daily life. Josephine Butler, an English social reformer who campaigned for women's rights, wrote to her son in 1896: "It occurred to me when this wonderful discovery could possibly be brought to bear upon the problem of the London fog! If light & vision could be brought into the heart of total darkness, could they not use the same power to bring light into the heart of a fog & turn darkness into daylight?"[8] Although Butler frames her response as a practical one, the slippage into metaphors of light and dark reflect a set of tropes that sprang up alongside X-rays and which we still use today: they shine light into darkness; they reveal truths; they will make the world a safer and more secure place.

Based in this belief, within weeks of Roentgen's discovery, border agents and customs officials in France were using X-rays to scan luggage and passengers.[9] On April 7, 1896, Eric Barrington, the Principal Private Secretary to the British Foreign Secretary Lord Salisbury, wrote to Sir Frank Lascelles, the British Ambassador to Germany, about a rumor:

> Monty Loftus, old Ld. Augustus's son, is undergoing a cure for lupus at Hamburgh. He overheard some Germans in the "Clinick" say that Roentgen rays were to be utilized by the . . . police for deciphering letters without opening them. No one knows what the capabilities of this fearful invention may be, but personally I doubt whether much could be made of handwriting on paper folded several times over. However I send you the rumour which may amuse you.[10]

Barrington was mostly correct in his assumption that the X-ray technology of 1896 would be incapable of reading folded letters, but his initial concerns echo the broader ones of the period. Would X-rays make secrets a thing of the past? Could people or empires exist without secrets? What were the limits of this new technology? Who would be allowed to wield it?

One of the greatest features of Roentgen's early work with X-rays was its accessibility. Roentgen never patented his discovery, believing it belonged to the world, nor did he invent anything new, perse. Rather, he engineered a device from readily available materials which were capable of producing X-rays. Then, he gave it away, publishing not only his discovery but also his process for making and operating his X-ray machine. His actions opened opportunities for many people outside traditional university systems to participate in the new and exciting scientific discovery. One such early innovator was a young Jewish-American woman named Elizabeth Fleischman.

Born in 1867 to Jewish-Austrian immigrants living in California, Fleischman did not complete high school, dropping out to work and support her family. She was entirely self-taught and not yet thirty in 1896, when she began working with X-rays. She soon opened her own professional X-ray clinic in San Francisco, the first of its kind in California, where she quickly gained a reputation for the spatial awareness and clarity of her X-ray images.

In 1898, with the Spanish-American War (April–August 1898) and subsequent Philippine-American War (1898–1902), the US Army shipped wounded soldiers from the Philippines to San Francisco, where many were X-rayed by Fleischman.

Her X-rays were praised for their clarity and precision which allowed doctors to extract bullets and shrapnel from soldiers without the need for additional exploratory procedures that put soldiers at risk for infections. So prominent was Fleischman, that the *San Francisco Chronicle* ran a full-page article on her, titled "The Woman Who Takes the Best Radiographs." The article showcased seven examples of her work including X-rays of bullet wounds in soldiers returning from the Philippines. Her most famous X-ray was of American soldier Private John Gretzer Jr. Although shot in the head, Gretzer lost consciousness for just a day and recovered with only slight paralysis to his right side. In their effort to understand his miraculous recovery, doctors requested Fleischman take the X-rays. Her images revealed that the bullet had lodged in the base of Gretzer's skull but posed no further threat to him. The article included a photograph of Gretzer alongside his X-ray, an uncanny image of life and almost-death.

Like many of the earliest innovators and adaptors of X-ray technology, Fleischman used her own hand as a test object to calibrate her machine before each use—a decision that would prove fatal. In 1904, only eight years after she opened her studio, Fleischman's right arm became cancerous from radiation poisoning and had to be amputated. She had taken some precautions in her practice, such as wearing rubber gloves and standing behind thick glass barriers when operating the machine, but these provided little protection against the radiation that she and other X-ray pioneers experienced. Never fully recovering her health, Fleischman died in August 1905. The *San Francisco Chronicle*, which had publicized her achievements only a few years earlier, titled her obituary "Death of a Famous Woman Radiographer," a final nod to Fleischman's work.

Early pioneers of X-ray technology bore the brunt of such discoveries and many of the first wave of innovators and scientists suffered the same fate as Fleischman. In the 1890s and early 1900s, it was common to have exposure times between twenty minutes to an hour—sometimes even two hours! The X-rays of this period were weaker and longer exposures created higher-quality images. The X-rays used in *Smith v. Grant*, for example, had exposure times of eighty minutes to produce the clearest images. Early X-ray innovators did notice burns and red rashes, but it took time to recognize the long-term dangers such exposures posed.

Even Thomas Edison, who had built his own X-ray machine only four days after reading about Roentgen's discovery, reported lingering vision problems after experimenting with X-rays. Initially enthralled with the new technology, Edison experimented with the portable fluoroscope, a device that allowed users to see their bones in real time. Viewers would place their hand on a wooden box that contained a vacuum tube emitting X-rays and peer through a fluoroscope, a fluorescent screen that projected a user's X-rays without the need to develop the images. When Edison, along with his assistant Clarence Dally, demonstrated the device at the 1896 National Electrical Exposition in New York, crowds swarmed to see it in action. The lure to see inside oneself was too great a temptation to resist.

Thousands of exposure hours caused Dally to suffer horrific burns, and ultimately, the painful carcinoma lesions necessitated the complete amputation of his left arm and part of his right. Working with invisible rays left visible damage on the body. Dally died in 1904, less than a year before Fleischman. *The New York Times* hailed him as a "martyr to science" with some claiming him to be the first casualty of X-rays.[11] Fearful after Dally's death, Edison ceased experimenting with X-rays. When questioned about his decision, he is reported to have said: "Do not talk to me about X-rays...I am afraid of them."[12] In his later years, suffering from poor health and abscesses in his teeth, Edison told his doctor that if his teeth were abscessed, he should extract them rather than use X-rays.

And it wasn't just the radiation that was dangerous. The film on which X-rays were made proved to be just as deadly. In 1929 at the Cleveland Clinic in Ohio, a fire broke out in the sub-basement room used to store X-ray films. At the time, X-ray film was made from a volatile and highly flammable cellulose-nitrate base. When burned, cellulose nitrate produces poisonous gases, including carbon monoxide, and once on fire, it is almost impossible to extinguish with water. Since the fire began in a sub-basement room, the odorless and tasteless poison gas was able to move unnoticed through the building's ventilation system. As the fire increased, explosions sent even greater volumes of gas through the vents. People outside the hospital heard the explosions and rushed to help, but they were quickly overcome by the toxic gases. In total, 123 people died. Remembered today as the Cleveland Clinic X-ray Fire of 1929, its exact cause was never determined, but its aftermath led to new guidelines for storing X-ray film and the creation of Safety X-ray Film, which uses a more stable cellulose-acetate base that does not produce poisonous gases when burned.

Like Prometheus, whom the gods punished for bringing fire down from the heavens, Roentgen also did not emerge unscathed. In the years following 1896, he was dogged by slanderous rumors that he had stolen the discovery from an assistant and, like an evil villain, was selling it to the highest bidder. There were also questions about scientific firsts. Before Roentgen, other physicists had unknowingly produced radiographic images, including Arthur Goodspeed in 1890 and Nikola Tesla in 1894. Roentgen's most vocal opponent, however, was the German physicist Philipp Lenard: "I am the mother of X-rays. Just as the mid-wife is not responsible for the mechanism of birth, so was Roentgen not responsible for the discovery of X-rays since all the groundwork had been prepared by me. Without me, the name of Roentgen would be unknown today."[13] Lenard claimed his own experiments had produced X-rays in 1892 and that he had shared his findings with Roentgen. Despite all these claims, no other scientist but Roentgen recognized the implications or significance of X-rays and what their discovery would mean for the world.

In 1901, Roentgen received the first Nobel Prize in Physics. He donated the prize money of 150,000 Swedish Krona (almost $1 million USD in 2024) to Naturforscher und Aerzte Gesellschaft, the Society of German Natural Scientists and Physicians, to support other scientists. In 1919, Roentgen retired; Anna Bertha died the same year after a long illness. On February 10, 1923, at the age of 78, Roentgen died from intestinal carcinoma, possibly stemming from his work with X-rays. He died in relative poverty, never profiting from his discovery, and even though he had not wanted to name X-rays after himself, the German word for X-ray, *der Roentgenstrahl*, commemorates his discovery still.

2 MANIA

"I'm built for the X-ray skirts and I'm going to wear 'em."

— BERTHA HANSCOM

From tulips and railways to The Beatles and Beanie Babies, manias are snapshots of human culture at a particular moment, revealing how new technologies, trends, or inventions shaped generations and sometimes changed the course of human history. X-rays changed almost every facet of human culture, and X-ray mania was evidence of a radical paradigm shift that X-rays instigated. When Roentgen published his discovery on January 1, 1896, the world changed irrevocably, and X-ray mania in equal parts questioned, celebrated, and revealed the world anew.

Almost immediately, "X-ray" became a marketing buzzword to sell products from liniment and headache tablets to stove polish and golf balls. These things had no real connection to X-rays, but companies and copywriters like those for X-ray's Renovator, a laundry detergent that promised to penetrate stains, understood the marketing appeal.

> The Roentgen Rays, the Roentgen Rays,
> What is this craze?
> The town's ablaze
> With the new phase
> Of X-ray's ways.
>
> I'm full of daze
> Shock and amaze
> For nowadays
> I hear they'll gaze
> Thro' cloak and gown—and even stays
> Those naughty, naughty Roentgen Rays.

—"X-actly So!"[1]

X-rays led to a new way of seeing and thinking about the world. Tongue-in-cheek poems and cartoons played upon themes of nakedness and exposure, but these satires spoke to real concerns for privacy, a concern that was magnified by the other great invention of 1895—film.

It's no coincidence that the language of X-rays—projection, image, screen—is shared with that of film. Roentgen's 1895 discovery occurred concurrently with the Lumière Brothers' work on early cinematography. At public fairs or theatrical shows, X-rays and the portable fluoroscope were displayed often alongside early films, linking the two discoveries in the public mind. In 1896, "Dr. McIntyre's X-ray Film," the first medical X-ray film, was created at the Glasgow Royal Infirmary and later shown at the London Royal Society in 1897. This two-minute film shows the muscles move inside a frog's leg as it extends and contracts; the valves of a heart open and close as it pumps blood; and stomach digestion as a solution of bismuth moves through it. In October 1897, less than two years after Roentgen's discovery, a 45-second silent film directed by English pioneer filmmaker George Albert Smith titled *The X-rays*, or *The X-ray Fiend*, was released.

The film opens with a couple seated on a bench against a black backdrop. They are fashionably dressed with the man in a suit and straw hat and the woman in late-Victorian dress with an elaborate hat and parasol. Flirtations are exchanged and the man clasps the woman's hand, kissing it periodically. Then, a second man in a dark suit appears to the right of screen. In his hands, he holds a white box outfitted with a telephoto-style lens, giving it the look of an 1890s image projector known as a magic lantern. On the side in black lettering, the word "X RAYS" appears. As he approaches the couple, he removes the lens cap. Using a jump shot (one of the first recorded jump shots in history), the film cuts between frames transforming the couple into a pair of skeletons.

With his bony legs bouncing, the man clutches the woman's hand even tighter as she attempts to pull away. The transformation lasts only thirteen seconds before the X-ray camera operator puts the lens cap back on and slowly backs

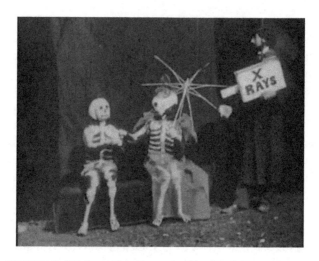

FIGURE 3 Still from *The X-rays*, or *The X-ray Fiend* (October 1897), directed by George Albert Smith, who also plays the X-ray camera operator. Smith's wife, Laura Bayley, plays the woman, and comedian Tom Green plays the man. Public domain.

out of the frame, ending the transformation. Returned to their normal forms, the man continues to grasp the woman's hand a few seconds longer before her expression turns to shock and she stands, pulling her hand away. The man kneels before her, his arms outstretched pleading, but she slaps him and walks out of the frame. His faced screwed up in displeasure, he sits on the bench, shoves his hat on his head, and pouts as the film ends.

A short but important film, *The X-rays* reveals how audiences in 1897 understood the relationship between the visual mediums of film and X-ray. George Albert Smith, the film's director, also plays the X-ray camera operator in a move that conflates film director with X-ray operator. Such doubling not only highlights the film director as voyeur, but also overlaps the nascent industries of cinematography and X-ray technology.

The two titles, *The X-rays* and *The X-ray Fiend*, create some ambiguity over tone. Are the X-rays being personified as fiends? Is the man holding the X-ray camera the fiend for his voyeuristic surveillance? Do the X-rays transform the lover into a fiend? Or, do they merely reveal his inner desire? He certainly seems more aggressively amorous in those thirteen seconds of transformation than before or after. What of the woman? Is she unaffected? The answers are unclear. What is clear is how the film portrays Victorian beliefs that X-rays were *active* beams with the ability to transform, and this theme appears frequently in early films about X-rays.

French filmmaker Georges Méliès, known for his groundbreaking early silent films *A Trip to the Moon* (1902) and *The Impossible Voyage* (1904) and for pioneering many special effect technologies, directed his own X-ray-inspired film *Les Rayons Roentgen*, or *A Novice at X-rays* (1898). This film is lost today, so we only have brief descriptions of its plot. It features a man visiting his doctor for an X-ray. Once the doctor activates the X-ray machine, the man unzips his skin and his skeleton steps out and begins moving about the room. The doctor then reverses the process, making the man whole again. Not feeling any better after the X-ray, the man refuses to pay the doctor. The film's conclusion is a bit murky, but most accounts suggest that the man attacks the X-ray machine which then explodes. Displaying the playful and surrealist themes typical of Méliès, the film highlights the misconception of X-rays as curative rather than diagnostic.

Other films drew upon real-life experiences such as Alice Guy-Blaché's *L'Utilité des Rayons X* (1898), in which border agents and customs officials use an X-ray fluoroscope to discover that a pregnant woman crossing the border is really a man smuggling contraband into the country. Some filmmakers embraced the psychological horror of X-rays, including Wallace McCutcheon's *The X-ray Mirror* (1899), in which a woman trying on hats in front of an X-ray mirror faints when she sees her skeleton, and Èmile Vardannes's *Un Ragno nel Cervello*, or *A Spider on the Brain* (1912), a film that can only be described as nightmare fuel, in which X-rays are used to locate a spider that has nested inside a person's brain.

The contribution of X-rays to the history of film and television does not end there. X-rays inspired one of the most recognized visual tropes—X-ray Sparks. The image occurs when a character receives a jolt of electricity, usually from lightning or an electrified wire, making the character's skeleton briefly visible through their body. The first alleged appearance of X-Ray Sparks was in a 1934 cartoon titled "The Discontented Canary," in which lightning strikes a cat causing its skeleton to glow from within. Filmmakers often employ the trope for comedic effect, such as in *Home Alone*

2: Lost in New York when the bumbling but loveable burglar Marv grabs onto faucet handles that Kevin has connected to an AC/DC arc welder. As Marv is electrocuted, his body is temporarily replaced with that of a skeleton (a slight variation on the trope). In other instances, X-ray Sparks create moments of real and metaphorical insight into a character.

During the Battle of Endor in *Return of the Jedi* (1983), when Darth Vader saves Luke, Vader lifts Emperor Palpatine over his head. As he does, Vader absorbs Palpatine's Force lightning, also known as dark rays. In brief flashes, the Force lightning illuminates Vader's skeleton, revealing the human and machine parts of his body. It fades as he throws Palpatine into the reactor core of the second Death Star. The X-ray Sparks give real and metaphorical glimpses into Vader's otherwise impenetrable character. They reveal the physical remnants of his humanity and signify his decision to betray the dark side and save Luke over himself. Even though Palpatine uses Force lightning to torture Luke, we never see Luke's skeleton. X-ray Sparks appear exclusively with Darth Vader.

Early filmmakers were not the only ones inspired by the horrific potential of X-rays. Writers of *fin-de-siècle* science fiction and Gothic literature also took note. George Griffith, an English science fiction writer, published one of the first literary works to respond to X-rays. In April 1896, *Pearson's Magazine* published Griffith's "A Photograph of the Invisible," a short story about X-rays and revenge. In Griffith's story, the jilted lover Denton exacts revenge on Edith, his ex-fiancée, with the help of his friend Professor Grantham, an amateur X-ray photographer. Together, they trick Edith into believing she is having her photograph taken in the newest style, unaware that she is receiving an X-ray. When Edith and her new husband receive the photograph, she gets a terrifying shock: "Above were her features . . . and, beneath all, sharp in outline and perfect in every hideous detail, a fleshless skull— her own skull—grinned at her through the transparent veil of flesh."[2] Gazing at her X-ray, Edith comes to believe "she is a skeleton, and that her clothing and skin and flesh are nothing more than transparent shadows which everybody can see through."[3] She suffers a nervous breakdown that sends her into an existential crisis over the nature of reality and her own corporeal existence. Ultimately, she withdraws from the world to live in isolation in a darkened room.

Apart from its misogynistic gaslighting of Edith, "A Photograph of the Invisible" captures the paradigmatic shifts in vision, identity, and reality that X-rays instigated. The timing of Roentgen's discovery coincided with Freud's 1895 publication *Studies on Hysteria*, a work of early psychoanalysis that examines the body's somatic responses to unconscious or repressed trauma. Griffith's story neatly combines the two. These ideas were also at the heart of another popular work inspired by X-rays: H.G. Wells's *The Invisible Man* (1897).

Wells's early science fiction tells the story of Griffin, a young scientist who feels ignored by society. Described by himself as a six-foot-tall albino with red eyes, Griffin feels invisible to his classmates and unacknowledged by his faculty. Believing himself intellectually superior to all men, Griffin is arrogant, impatient, and violent with those around him, a classic example of Nietzsche's Übermensch, a superior human or a superman. Using his knowledge of physics and optical density, Griffin develops a procedure by which he is able "to lower the refractive index of a substance, solid or liquid, to that of air," effectively turning the matter invisible.[4] He tests this procedure first on a white pillowcase and a white cat before attempting the experiment on himself. It is Griffin's albinism, a genetic condition by which a person's body produces little to no melanin, that makes it possible for him to lower the refractive index of his body and turn invisible. But Griffin is rash and impulsive, and he turns himself invisible with no forethought for how he will turn back.

Griffin discovers that invisibility is not the superpower he had imagined. For starters, to be invisible, he must be entirely nude, and when the novel opens, it's February in England. Griffin finds that being invisible does not suspend the body's other processes: undigested food is visible in his stomach; when his feet get dirty, people can see them; dogs can smell him; his transparent eyelids make it impossible to sleep; and because it is winter and he is naked, he is constantly sick, and his loud sneezes give him away.

When we first meet Griffin, he has been invisible for several months and has retreated to a small English village, seeking solitude to experiment and find a way back to himself. When he arrives in the village, his appearance draws unwanted attention immediately:

> He was wrapped up from head to foot, and the brim of his soft felt hat hid every inch of his face but the shiny tip of his nose. . . . he wore big blue spectacles with side-lights, and had a bushy side-whisker over his coat collar that completely hid his cheeks and face. . . . all his forehead above his blue glasses was covered by a white bandage, and that another covered his ears, leaving not a scrap of his face exposed excepting only his pink, peaked nose. It was bright, pink, and shiny just as it had been at first.[5]

Griffin's bandaged face seems overwhelmed by his prostheses; the shiny nose, the blue spectacles, and the abundant side-whiskers, which serve to make him visible, emphasize the plasticity of the human form. His relationship to his prostheses, however, is tenuous. He wears them out of necessity. He needs other people to perceive him as a person, even though to the villagers his appearance is more akin to a grotesque assemblage of objects rather than a human being. The dark irony of Griffin's predicament—an invisible man who must make his invisibility invisible so that he can blend into a crowd once again—yes, this dark irony is part of Wells's humor, an extension of the novel's message: an invisible man is an absurd thing.

In chapter seven of *The Invisible Man*, "The Unveiling of the Stranger," Griffin reaches his breaking point with the

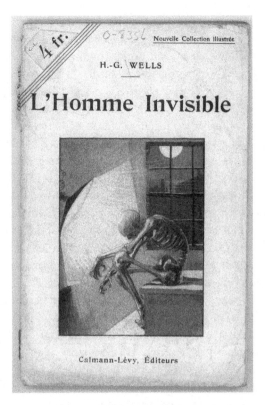

FIGURE 4 1912 French edition of *L'Homme Invisible*. The cover evokes the idea of X-rays through rays of light illuminating a skeleton. The earliest vacuum tubes used in generating X-rays were called "X-ray lamps." Courtesy of the Kenneth Spencer Research Library, University of Kansas.

villagers' curiosity and gossip. In a pique of anger in the village pub, he removes his prosthetic nose, handing it to an unsuspecting woman, and begins to unwind his bandages. The villagers' reaction is one of shock: "It was worse than anything. . . . They were prepared for scars, disfigurements, tangible horrors, but *nothing!* . . . . For the man who stood there shouting some incoherent explanation was a solid gesticulating figure up to the coat-collar . . . and then—nothingness, no visible thing at all!"[6] Wells's story not only brings to light the pragmatic problems with invisibility, but it also reveals the paradox of an invisible man. With the removal of his bandages, Griffin removes any semblance of a human form, revealing a nothingness that transcends the physical to the ontological: is an invisible man still a man?

After removing his prostheses and bandages, we find Griffin trying to persuade us that he exists at all: "The fact is I'm all here . . . I'm invisible. . . . I am."[7] His first statement, "The fact is I'm all here," is undercut by his invisibility. Perhaps recognizing the contradictory coupling of invisibility with the assertion that he is *here*, he tries again: "I'm invisible." This statement is problematic as the predicate through which he identifies himself effectively erases him. His last attempt is assertion: "I am." But "I am" by itself is a claim without evidence. It echoes the latter half of Descartes famous first principle *cogito, ergo sum*, or "I think, therefore I am."[8] The invisible man's final claim of "I am," or *ego sum*, calls himself into presence as a subject, an *ego*. In Barbara Johnson's words, however, "Nothing Descartes writes…proves that the being, whose existence he had demonstrated, was human."[9] Without a visible human body, the Invisible Man dissolves into pure ego. He is unable to prove his existence, his humanity. Without a predicate, he has become an unknown. He has become X.

What was perceived as a potentially utopian existence has turned nightmare. Griffin's invisibility has not freed him from the burden of a human body or the structures of modern civilization as he imagined. In the final chapter, unable to communicate and cut off from other men, Griffin determines to enact a new Reign of Terror, a modern anarchy. In response, a mob hunts him down, corners him, and beats him to death. As he dies, Griffin slowly regains his visible form:

> First came the little white nerves, a hazy grey sketch of a limb, then the glassy bones and intricate arteries, then the flesh and skin, first a faint fogginess, and then growing rapidly dense and opaque. . . . His hands were clenched, his eyes wide open, and his expression was one of anger and dismay. 'Cover his face!' said a man. 'For Gawd's sake, cover that face.'[10]

Only in death and only for a moment does Griffin become truly visible, before the crowd reacts with horror and hides his body from sight. Are they reacting to his appearance or to the physical evidence of their own savagery? Wells lets us decide. Throughout *The Invisible Man*, Wells takes up the metaphor of X-rays as tools of revelation and self-knowledge, but the final scene is a warning: we might not like what we find.

While writers and filmmakers, such as Wells and Méliès, imagined the creative potential of X-rays, public exhibitions held across America, Britain, and Europe in 1896 and 1897 allowed people to experience the reality of X-rays for themselves. The public's response was paradoxical, an ebb and flow between curiosity and confusion, fear and fascination, but what was frightful in 1896—public exposure—became fashionable in 1913.

Imported from Paris, sheer clothing, known as X-ray skirts, was a mini-mania in 1913. Prudish and misogynistic American newspapers expressed their moral outrage with headlines such as "X-ray Gown Starts a Riot" and "X-ray Skirts Break Up Home of Millionaire." Upon filing for divorce from her 60-year-old millionaire husband, Bertha Hanscom, 30 years old, declared: "My husband is an old fossil . . . I'm built for the X-ray skirts and I'm going to wear 'em. He doesn't like them, but I don't care. Wait until I get my divorce and I'll make his eyes pop."[11] You go and get it, Bertha!

There was even a popular revue song. "In Your X-ray Gown" (1913) tells the story of Daisy, a young woman with a passion for clothes and her X-ray gown. As she walks about town, she meets different men who sing the chorus:

In the X-ray gown you're wearing,
You're rather daring, you're rather daring.

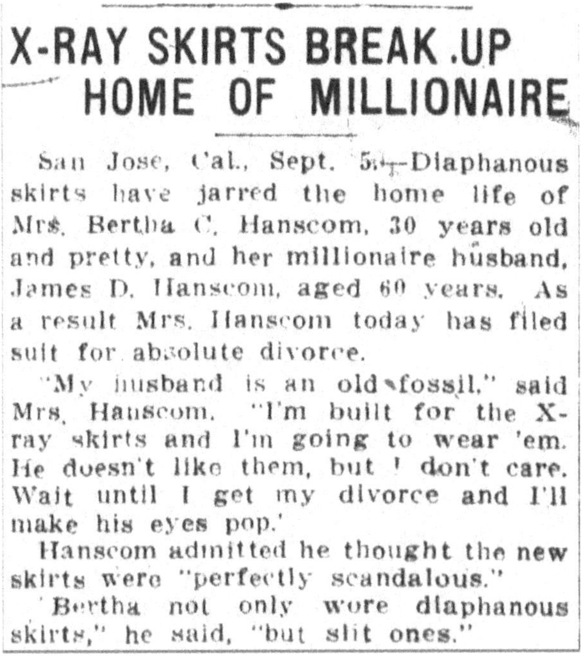

X-RAY SKIRTS BREAK UP HOME OF MILLIONAIRE

San Jose, Cal., Sept. 5.—Diaphanous skirts have jarred the home life of Mrs. Bertha C. Hanscom, 30 years old and pretty, and her millionaire husband, James D. Hanscom, aged 60 years. As a result Mrs. Hanscom today has filed suit for absolute divorce.

"My husband is an old fossil," said Mrs. Hanscom. "I'm built for the X-ray skirts and I'm going to wear 'em. He doesn't like them, but I don't care. Wait until I get my divorce and I'll make his eyes pop.'

Hanscom admitted he thought the new skirts were "perfectly scandalous."

'Bertha not only wore diaphanous skirts," he said, "but slit ones."

FIGURE 5 "X-Ray Skirts Break Up Home of Millionaire." Published in the *Oregon Daily Journal*, September 5, 1913.

I admire your style,
And I'd simply love to watch you all the while.
In your new transparent costume
You'll capture the town;
It's rather 'warm',

But you show 'good form'
In your X ray gown.[12]

For Daisy and Bertha, X-ray clothing is empowering and feminine. By making women's bodies visible, X-ray clothing gives women control, and women today still use sheer or translucent clothing to make powerful statements about their bodies, sexuality, and women's roles within social and cultural hierarchies. Sheer clothing is almost never out of style thanks to fashion houses and celebrities such as Beyoncé (in Dolce & Gabbana, 2023 Oscars party), Jennifer Lopez (in Versace, 2000 VMAs), and Florence Pugh (in Valentino, 2022 Haute Couture fashion show), all of whom have worn sheer gowns to high-profile media events. Public reaction today is as mixed as it was in 1913—titillation and awe mixed with outrage and censorship.

From the first publication of Anna Bertha's hand and the short film *The X-ray Fiend*, voyeurism and the objectification of women's bodies has been central to the story of X-rays. In the 1920s, chiropractic organizations began holding "posture contests." These were beauty contests with an added emphasis on posture and deportment. The winners became known as Posture Queens. In 1955, contest organizers in Michigan added a new component—X-rays. The straightest spine wins. The judge-chiropractors examined contestants alongside their X-rays.

By 1957, national and international posture contests were also including contestants' X-rays as part of their judgements. The *Chiropractic Economics* reported "Posture Contests are BIG Business" because they brought glamour and media attention to an unsexy industry.[13] American and World Posture Queens were treated like celebrities, appearing on *The Tonight Show* with Jack Paar and receiving invitations from President Johnson to visit the White House. Despite their success and popularity, posture contests were discontinued in the 1970s, possibly due to the counterculture movements of the 1960s and the women's rights movement. Other reports suggest that increasing concerns over unnecessary radiation exposure had cast a negative light on the events.

As people became accustomed to the new technology, they began finding new ways to solve old problems. For example, the shoe fluoroscope, also known as the Foot-O-Scope in England or the X-ray Shoe Fitter in the US, was a non-medical device found in shoe stores and department stores from the 1920s to the 1960s. The shoe fluoroscope was a three-foot-tall rectangular box with a viewing window in the top and two arched openings in the bottom for the user's feet. Designed for sales associates and shoppers, these fluoroscopes allowed users to see how their feet fit into a pair of shoes. I imagine parents of small children loved the convenience of such machines, never mind the radiation. The US military also used the machines to measure soldiers' boots, and orthopedic doctors used them to diagnose foot pain. Growing concerns over unnecessary radiation exposure caused the machines to be removed in the 1960s. By 1970, 33 states in the US had banned them entirely. Paradoxically, the machines were causing the very thing they were designed to prevent—foot problems.

X-ray mania, like other manias, cooled after a few years, but it left a lasting impression that we can still see. Like their predecessors selling X-ray headache tablets and X-ray golf balls, modern advertisers still use X-rays in marketing campaigns for things that have nothing to do with X-rays. In 2003, the Got Milk? campaign offered people the opportunity to appear in a television commercial. The cost of entry? Their X-rays. Using the tagline "Got Bones?," the Got Milk? campaign asked people to submit their X-rays with the claim: "Your bones could make you famous." I guess people worried about medical privacy a lot less back then.

In 2016, Mercedes Benz suggested their new powerful headlights were akin to X-rays. Ads showed the headlights shining through the bodies of deer on the roadway, implying that the lights would give drivers X-ray-like vision while driving at night. In 2018, to combat the claims that they used fake chicken, KFC used X-rays of chicken legs and wings with the tagline "Real Chicken." Not to be outdone, Burger King in 2019 used X-rays of dislocated jaws from allegedly real customers to advertise the size of their Whopper and Mega Stacker sandwiches. Each X-ray included the tagline: "We warned you it was big." In 2021, the London-based advertising company Karmarama designed a holiday gift-wrapping paper that showed gift receivers an X-ray of the object inside. Named X-wrap and "made to throw gift guessers off their game," customers could choose between an X-ray of a reindeer sweater, a toilet brush, an engagement ring, or a pair of headphones. So come the holiday season, what looked like a gifted toilet brush might be an expensive bottle of wine.

By their very nature, X-rays lead to lots of opportunities for visual gags that depend on visual confusion or misperceptions. While some advertisers capitalize on this feature for profit, other advertisers have used it to promote change. In 2015, the American nonprofit organization Ad Council designed a television ad campaign titled "Love Has No Labels." Filmed on Valentine's Day 2015, the television spot opens near the Santa Monica Pier in California with a crowd watching a pair of skeletons embrace and kiss on a large fluoroscope-style screen. After they kiss, the skeletons walk to either side of the screen and peek around to reveal themselves to the audience. Shots of the crowd's reactions show surprise, excitement, and encouragement, as each subsequent couple dances or embraces before revealing themselves to the audience. The couples' identities are diverse, showing a range of races, ages, religions, and bodies. The tagline "Love has no labels" is adapted to reflect each couple: "Love has no gender"; "Love has no race"; "Love has no disability"; "Love has no religion"; "Love has no age." The campaign uses X-rays to promote community and equality, and challenges viewers' unconscious biases. It sends the message that, when it comes to love, we are the same, you x me. The surface differences are just that—surface.

Humans process a lot of information with our eyes, so any new technology that affects vision and our comprehension of the world brings with it a level of excitement different from other technologies. X-ray mania was, in part, a series of imaginative responses to the impacts that X-rays could and did have on human life, but it was also about the sheer excitement for a discovery that suddenly and startingly made the world anew.

3 VISION

"It doesn't take X-ray vision to see you are up to no good"

— SUPERMAN

Vision is regarded widely as the most valuable of the human senses, and Roentgen's discovery promised to push the boundaries of vision beyond its physical limits, transforming the impossible into possibility. Reports of second sight, clairvoyance, and extrasensory perception (ESP) date back to the sixteenth century, but those claiming such abilities were viewed as disturbed, divinely inspired, or even demonic. In 1896, the discovery of a wavelength of light capable of seeing through objects radically altered people's perceptions of what was possible in the natural world. After 1895, people possessed of naturally-occurring X-ray vision became, for the first time, a plausible reality.

With approximately 20 million deaths in the First World War (1914–1918) and 50 million deaths from the 1918 flu pandemic, survivors and bereaved families turned in increasing numbers to Spiritualism and the Spiritualist movement for solace. A divisive religious movement, spiritualists believed that the living could make contact with departed souls through seances and communicate with the dead through table rapping, automatic writing, and spirit photography. The X-ray, which offered to extend human sight beyond its physical boundaries, was incorporated into spiritualist practices with the belief that X-rays could capture images of souls. It is in this period that *Scientific American*, a well-respected magazine then as it is now, began a competition in 1922 asking for proof of psychic or supernatural abilities. The winner would receive $2,500; over $45,000 in 2024. The judges included scientists, psychic experts, a psychologist, an occult writer, and Harry Houdini. Famous worldwide for his own stunts, performances, and sleight-of-hand magic, Houdini devoted himself to exposing fraudulent mystic seers and mediums, especially those that took advantage of the grieving and the vulnerable.

In 1924, the year after Roentgen's death, Harry Houdini published a forty-page pamphlet titled *HOUDINI exposes the tricks used by the BOSTON MEDIUM 'MARGERY' to win the $2500 prize offered by the Scientific American. Also a complete exposure of ARGAMASILLA the famous Spaniard who baffled noted Scientists of Europe and America, with his claim to X-RAY VISION*. Of the two exposures Houdini offered in his 1924 pamphlet, Margery's is the more famous, in part because Houdini was never able in his lifetime to prove conclusively that she was a fraud. In 1924, however, Houdini had his keen eyes also set on Joaquin Maria Argamasilla, the "Spaniard with X-ray Eyes." At only nineteen years old, Argamasilla had gained an international reputation for his ability to read through objects: "This phenomenal mystifier essayed to perform or accomplish the impossible: he makes claim to a power of supernormal vision, X-ray eyes and a penetrating brain."[1] When they met in New York, Argamasilla came with letters written by "noted scientists of Spain who attested" that the young Spaniard had "proved conclusively to their satisfaction *that he could read through metal*."[2] Houdini put him to the test.

Argamasilla traveled with two small unpainted metal boxes, which he invited spectators to place objects, such as coins or calling cards. Argamasilla claimed he could see through the metal and he would announce what he saw. The main event of Argamasilla's act was his reading the time on a closed-face pocket watch placed into one of the boxes. In front of an audience, Houdini explains, Argamasilla would ask for a pocket watch with a cover over the watch face. As the participant sets the watch to a random time, Argamasilla blindfolds himself by placing cotton wool over his eyes and then wrapping his handkerchief, which has been pre-folded, around his head. He then asks for the watch to be placed in his right hand, face up with the case closed. He holds the watch for a moment, sometimes lifting his left hand to his temple or furrowing his brow, before holding the watch up to the audience to show it remains closed. Then, he places the watch into the box. After a few moments of suspense,

Argamasilla announces the time set on the watch, which he confirms by pulling out the watch and revealing it to the crowd.

In his pamphlet, Houdini exposes the trick as nothing more than sleight-of-hand stage magic. When receiving the watch, the blind-folded Argamasilla performs a sweeping hand movement that allows him to slide the cover back ever so slightly. At the same moment, Argamasilla either furrows his brow or touches his left hand to his blindfold, either of which shifts the blindfold enough for him to look down and glimpse the time before he presents the watch to the audience and places it into the box. Houdini elaborates that when he gave Argamasilla a watch with a tricky cover, he was unable to perform his supernatural feat. Houdini concludes by claiming that he has performed the same trick with success: "Since witnessing his performance I have presented the watch trick and so far, no one has been able to detect the movement unless knowing, before-hand, the trick of opening and closing the watch."[3] After his encounter with Houdini, Argamasilla never performed in public again.

Despite the exposure of Argamasilla, there were other reports of people with X-ray vision. Kuda Bux, a Pakistani magician, performed feats of X-ray vision to crowds from the 1930s until the 1970s. Captured on film by British Pathé in 1938 (and now available to view on YouTube), Bux's method included placing cotton over his closed eyes and then bandaging his entire head, giving him a resemblance to Wells's Invisible Man. In the short documentary *The*

Man with X-ray Eyes!, Bux performs a series of tests while blindfolded: copying out a sentence, lighting a man's cigarette, and walking through a small obstacle course, all in front of a crowd of spectators who seem delighted with the performance. Bux claimed he could control his eyesight through his nostrils; so, when his head was wrapped, he insisted his nostrils must remain clear. Skeptics claimed that Bux could see by looking down the sides of his nose. Unlike Argamasilla, Bux never had to contend with Houdini, who had died in 1926 before Bux rose to prominence.

In the years that followed, Bux gained popularity as "The Man with X-ray Eyes." He even inspired writer Roald Dahl. Published in 1977, Dahl's story "The Wonderful Story of Henry Sugar" follows the wealthy Henry Sugar who reads a doctor's report about an Indian patient who calls himself "The Man Who Can See Without His Eyes." Sugar then embarks on a journey to learn the man's secret meditation methods that allow him to see without the use of his eyes. The man in Dahl's story was inspired by Bux, who also claimed to have learned his skill from a yogi. Bux continued to perform right up until his death in 1981.

Let's be honest. Stories like Argamasilla's and Bux's are rather dull. Even if they could see through objects, they performed only parlor tricks. Where is the action? Where is the drama and power that X-ray vision promises? Well, when Argamasilla and Bux achieved recognition, X-rays had an image problem. In the 1930s, people were curious about X-rays, but they were also afraid—and rightly so! By the 1930s, the first wave of X-ray scientists and amateurs had died, their deaths often the result of their work. Roentgen himself had died from a form of intestinal cancer, probably caused by radiation exposure. Radiation pioneers, such as Marie Curie, and new technologies were making X-rays safer, but even Curie died in 1934 from aplastic anemia, likely the result of excessive radiation exposure. Famously, Marie Curie was buried in a lead-lined coffin, and her laboratory notebooks, which are stored in lead boxes at the Bibliothèque Nationale de France in Paris, are so radioactive that researchers wishing to examine them must wear protective clothing and sign a liability waiver. In the 1930s, it was obvious from the body of evidence—and from the bodies themselves—that a human with real X-ray vision was an impossibility. The human body simply could not survive it. Who could? The answer: an alien.

Olga Mesmer first appeared in 1937 in a comic strip titled "The Astounding Adventures of Olga Mesmer, the Girl with the X-ray Eyes," published in *Spicy Mystery Stories*. Olga's story opens with her mother, Queen Margot, forced

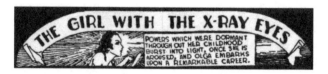

FIGURE 6 The title logo for Olga Mesmer, the *Girl with the X-ray Eyes*, first published in 1937 in the pulp magazine *Spicy Mystery Stories*. Artist unknown. Public domain via Wikipedia Commons.

to flee Venus, her home planet where she rules over the underground realm. On Earth, Queen Margot falls in love with and marries American scientist Dr. Hugo Mesmer. Mesmer, whose name alludes to Franz Mesmer, the father of hypnosis, conducts experiments on the now-pregnant Queen Margot using his patented "soluble X-rays." When she awakens from the experiment, Margot discovers that she has X-ray vision. Looking around the room for Hugo, she finds she can see through the wall, but on the other side is Hugo with another woman. In a fit of rage and jealousy, Margot kills Hugo with her X-ray vision. After giving birth to her daughter Olga, Margot returns to Venus, abandoning the half-human half-alien Olga on Earth to be raised by Rankin, her Venus-born guardian and protector. When Olga comes of age, her X-ray vision and superhuman strength begin to manifest, and through her adventures, Olga learns to harness her powers to protect the innocent, fight crime, and rescue those in need.

In illustrations, Olga is scantily clad, her dress often ripped and always slipping off her shoulders, a garter belt sometimes visible around one thigh. We don't need X-ray vision to see Olga's nearly-naked body. Repeatedly rejecting men's advances, Olga is desirable but unattainable. She is exotic but familiar, powerful but controlled, heroic but humble. Olga demonstrates X-ray vision can be used in the service of justice and truth.

If Margot embodies X-ray vision as raw, alien, and dangerous, Olga embodies it as controlled and humane, perhaps because Olga herself is half-human. Despite her many heroic deeds, chastity, and humility, however, Olga is still a woman—and a powerful woman is dangerous. To view the world through the X-ray vision of a woman in 1938, even a half-alien one, would reveal a world of injustices and inequities proliferated by men, a world possibly beyond redemption. In the hands of women, X-ray vision threatened masculinity. In the hands of men, it reinforced it.

It's probably no surprise then that just over a year after it began, Olga Mesmer's story ended. Readers, it seemed, didn't want a woman with superstrength, much less one with X-ray vision. In the final installments published in October 1938, Olga saves Rodney, a young human man, by giving him a blood transfusion. In the process, she transfers her powers to him. Together, Olga and Rodney travel to Venus to restore her mother's throne. And there, Olga remains.

In 1938, with rising tensions in Europe, American readers wanted a superhero that reflected the strength of American morality and the honesty of American values. And in June 1938, four months prior to Olga's departure to Venus, they got it. A new superhero, the last of his kind, born with superhero strength and X-ray vision arrived on Earth. With his wholesome charm, good looks, and, most importantly, masculinity, Superman arrived to save mankind. There was no room on Earth for "The Girl with the X-ray Eyes."

Created by Jerry Siegel and Joe Shuster, Superman first appeared in June 1938 in *Action Comics #1*, but the first instance of his X-ray vision wouldn't come until September

1939 in issue #18. In its first print appearance, Superman uses his X-ray vision to spy on criminals through a brick wall. The first onscreen appearance of his X-ray vision came two years later in November 1941 in *The Mechanical Monsters*, a short animated film released by Paramount. In it, Superman uses his X-ray vision to rescue Lois Lane after she is taken hostage by an inventor's army of robots. Animators Steve Muffati and George Germanetti illustrated Superman's X-ray vision as light-gray flickering rays that emit from his eyes. *The Mechanical Monsters* also includes the very first instance of Clark Kent using a telephone booth to change into Superman, a feature that Siegel and Shuster would begin incorporating into the comic in 1942.

In keeping with the interests in nuclear energy science of the 1940s and 1950s, Superman's X-ray vision changes in 1949. In "The Man of Steel's Super Manhunt" *Superman #59* (July 1949), Superman travels to the North Atlantic in search of the man responsible for planting a bomb in Metropolis. Looking at a glacier, he is surprised to discover that he cannot see through it. He lands on a solution, though not a very eco-conscious one: "by turning on the full strength of my X-ray powers, I can use them to **melt** that oversize block of ice!"[4] And, using the "tremendous heat of his x-ray vision," Superman melts the glacier—only to discover that what blocked his vision was not the ice, but a lead tunnel built underneath the glacier. As in real life, lead is the only material capable of blocking X-rays. The term "heat vision" wouldn't be used officially until

1961, but in 1949, in its first appearance, it is a byproduct of Superman's X-ray vision.

In *Action Comics #227* (April 1957), titled "The Man with the Triple X-ray Eyes," Superman finds his X-ray vision has tripled in power, leaving him unable to control it. He crafts a pair of glasses made from solid lead, which block both his regular and X-ray vision. Unable to use his eyes and reliant only on his super hearing, Superman must learn to navigate the world anew with the help of a guide dog. Most of the issue is taken up with bad guys thinking they can trick Superman because he can't see them; they are of course wrong. In the conclusion, scientists uncover that Superman might be receiving extra radiation from a strange comet passing between Earth and the sun. Using his enhanced X-ray vision, Superman opens his eyes and expends the extra energy into the comet destroying it and regaining control. The final frame shows Superman giving his seeing-eye dog to a man who is blind. The man thanks him for how he has handled his temporary blindness and represented the blind community. Meant to serve as disability representation, it is an awkward moment since Superman is never actually blind. Readers would have to wait until the debut of Stan Lee's *Daredevil* in 1964 for a superhero who is blind.

While most people know about Superman's X-ray vision, only devoted fans will know that his power predates his creation. Siegel and Shuster did not do many interviews together, but in August 1983 in *Nemo: The Classic Comics Library #2*, the creators offered insight into the origins of

Superman and his famous abilities. In the interview, they discuss their early love of science fiction, especially the works of H.G. Wells, and the first comic strips they created together. One of those strips, Siegel says, was "about two pals who own some sort of mechanism which enables them to peer anywhere in the world, through walls or anything, and listen in on what gangsters are saying, and then get busy scotching the villainy. In a way, that was a forerunner of Superman's supervision and X-ray vision, only done with a mechanism. I don't remember the title—*Ralph* something."[5] Regrettably, no drawings of this earlier comic survive. Even so, Siegel and Shuster were clearly thinking about X-rays and X-ray vision long before they created Superman.

It's not known if Siegel and Shuster ever read *Spicy Mystery Series*, where Olga Mesmer appeared, but they were avid readers of the science fiction magazine *Amazing Stories*, which in 1931 serialized *Seeds of Life*, a novel by John Taine, the pseudonym for American writer Eric Temple Bell. In *Seeds of Life*, Taine explores the ability of X-rays to transform the human body. The novel follows Neils Bork, a laboratory assistant who is described as stocky, slovenly, and an alcoholic. One night in a drunken rage and with the intent of ending his life, Bork uses some experimental X-ray equipment to send over twenty million volts into his body, but an error on Bork's part prevents it from killing him. Instead, the energy transforms his mind and body, enhancing his mental acuity and turning his physique into that of a body builder—a superman. Taine's story rewrites the narrative of X-rays.

Instead of being dangerous to the human body, X-rays transform Bork into a better version of himself, making him fit, strong, and physically confident. Taine's novel reflects a growing change in the public's perception of X-rays.

In the 1930s, Olga Mesmer and Superman were putting imaginary X-ray vision into the service of public good, but something similar was also happening with real X-rays. During this period, outbreaks of tuberculosis were widespread across the United States, Britain, and Europe. With a chest X-ray, however, infected patients could be identified, quarantined, and treated. X-rays to the rescue! Starting in the 1930s and continuing into the 1960s, national chest X-ray campaigns were organized with buses and vans converted into mobile X-ray units reminiscent of the Little Curies from the First World War. In them, X-ray technicians and medical staff traveled the countryside offering free diagnostics to people in cities and rural communities.

To promote the campaign and demonstrate how easy and painless getting an X-ray was, celebrities and characters such as Lucille Ball and Santa Claus were featured in ad campaigns for tuberculosis screenings. Advertisements emphasized that chest X-rays could give one confidence in one's health. One such poster produced in Britain in the 1940s features a cartoon mother duck with two small ducklings set against a bright sunshine yellow background. Above their heads is the word **CONFIDENCE**, and below them: "In Your Future. Have Your Chest X-Rayed. Visit the Mass Radiography Unit Coming to this Area." The message wasn't exactly subtle: if you wanted to be confident that you weren't a carrier of a highly contagious and deadly disease, get a chest X-ray. Only X-rays could give you "confidence in your future."

Another American poster featured a muscular, bare-chested man, his hands poised above his hips à la Superman. Above him, the headline: "'*Healthy looks*' can hide TUBERCULOSIS." Below him: "the X-RAY will show it before *you* know it." The poster even includes a chest X-ray with red arrows pointing towards spots on the image, presumably evidence of inflammation or tubercles (nodular lesions in the lungs indicative of tuberculosis). X-rays could not prevent tuberculosis, but they could make it visible. The message of this poster is two-fold: one, even the healthiest individuals can be infected, and two, X-rays can reveal secrets that the body is keeping. This type of public health messaging relies not on confidence, but on fear: you might be sick and might not even know it. We see similar rhetoric used today in screening campaigns for everything from colon cancer to Covid.

In the 1940s, equating *clean* and *healthy* with *seeing* was central to tuberculosis campaigns, and X-rays were responsible, in part, for creating a clean and healthy world. This rhetoric filtered into other arenas of daily life. X-ray vision goes domestic! In 1912, Bessie Littleton, wife of Corning glass engineer Jesse Littleton, wanted to bake a cake, but her ceramic cake pan had cracked in the too-hot oven. Jesse gave his wife half of a battery jar made from a glass called Nonex, a thick but clear glass designed to be durable

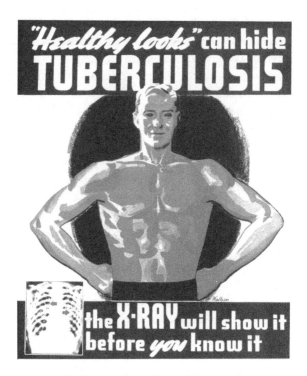

FIGURE 7 National Tuberculosis Association poster ca. 1935. Courtesy of the National Library of Medicine. Used by permission of the American Lung Association, www.lung.org.

in high temperatures. Using the half-jar, Bessie was able to bake a perfect cake, appreciative that she could monitor the cake's progress through the glass and noting that it cooked much quicker. Inspired, Jesse took the Nonex glass back to his laboratory and redesigned it, making it larger and more food safe. The first dish Corning created from this new glass was a pie dish. Pie + Nonex = Pyrex.

In its ad campaigns of the 1940s, Pyrex used its transparency as its main selling point. "When it's Pyrex Ware, you can <u>see</u> it's clean" reads a 1948 ad equating transparency with cleanliness. Another ad shows two children doing the dishes. The boy holds up a Pyrex glass tray to his face and peers through it: "It IS clean—you can SEE its clean—it's PYREX ware!" reads the ad copy. If we cannot give ourselves X-ray vision, we can do the next best thing—we can make a transparent world. Pyrex, Cellophane (invented in 1908), and Saran Wrap (first sold in 1953) were all designed with transparency in mind. In *X-ray Architecture*, Beatriz Colomina extends the transparency of household objects to mid-century glass houses: "The ability to see through material challenged all assumption and social protocols about privacy and psychological well-being and therefore all architectural concepts of shelter and comfort. . . . Just as the X-ray exposes the inside of the body to the public eye, the modern building exposed its interior."[6]

In the 1940s and 1950s, X-rays had proven that they could shine a light into all kinds of darkness. X-rays could save people from disease, resolve pain, and create a cleaner world. X-rays could also speak for those too young or unable to speak for themselves. In 1962, German-American doctor C. Henry Kempe coined the term "battered child syndrome." Like the creators of Superman, Jerry Siegel and Joe Shuster, Kempe was also from a Jewish family. In 1939, at age 17, he and his family fled Germany for America. Trained as a physician and pediatrician, Kempe worked at the University of Colorado as Chair of the Pediatrics Department.

In 1962, Kempe and two colleagues published "The Battered Child Syndrome" in the *Journal of the American Medical Association*. In their paper, Kempe and his colleagues described the uses of X-rays in children under the age of three who are unable to express their experiences: "To the informed physician, the bones tell a story the child is too young or too frightened to tell."[7] X-rays can reveal old injuries healed or new injuries that are in the process of healing, both of which can be invisible to the eye. Central to this work is the ability of physicians and technicians to *read* X-rays. As with all forms of reading though, interpretation is subjective and can be influenced by outside factors. Some practitioners were simply unwilling to believe that such cruelty and abuse, from broken limbs to fractured skulls, could be enacted on infants and small children, but such cases pointed to the critical need for intervention with medical imaging. X-rays helped bring awareness of child abuse into the larger social agenda because images of such trauma are persuasive. Seeing is believing.

The ability to diagnose such cases, however, is dependent on the reading of the X-rays. To those untrained, reading an X-ray can seem akin to modern divination with the radiologist as a mystic seer. As with any act of reading, X-rays can be misread, misinterpreted, or even misused. Even the X-rays themselves are not infallible. Images can contain shadows that falsely influence one's interpretation, or they can be distorted leading to false conclusions, as in the case of Tutankhamen. In the 1960s, medical professionals invited social workers to work alongside them to identify the signs of non-accidental injuries indicative of battered child syndrome. The move was radical because it coupled the ability to read X-rays—a kind of X-ray vision—with an ability to detect truth. In such cases, X-ray images are presented as irrefutable evidence of crimes against children. Radiologists become detectives and crime stoppers. They become (super) heroes.

Olga Mesmer, Superman, and radiologists, however, have limitations to their X-ray vision. What might unlimited X-ray vision reveal about the unseen parts of our world? This question was first asked in 1896 by French writer Charles Recolin in his short story "Le Rayon X." In it, surgeon-scientist Dr. Cornelius Schwanthaler discovers a liquid that when injected into the eye can give the user X-ray vision. Schwanthaler injects it into his left eye only, retaining normal vision in his right.

At first Schwanthaler is thrilled with his ability: "To see inside everything, to penetrate the very center of matter, to scrutinize the framework that sustains the human membrane and perhaps discover, in those depths, the secret of the soul and the prime movement of thought was a double dream of medicine and philosophy."[8] When he attends a ball, however, he finds he cannot appreciate the beauty of the dancers when he can see their skeletons at work beneath their forms. A trip to the countryside is unsettling—"the leafless colorless trees, loomed up like the tentacles of an octopus"— and his fiancée turns into "a frail skeleton . . . its tibias bumping together, with a gross stomach wobbling in front of it."[9] Horrified by what he sees, he flees. Away from town, Schwanthaler comes to the conclusion that "Ecclesiastes was right! . . . Whoever increases knowledge increases sorrow. God has retained the worst part for himself: the truth, which is sad. He has left us beauty, illusion and hope. And I have refused the role allotted to human beings, which was that of happiness."[10] In his grief and rage, he tears out his left eye, leaving him with only his right eye, the good eye, the eye that sees beauty.

A minister as well as a writer, Recolin captures a recurrent question asked in the aftermath of Roentgen's discovery: With the power of X-rays, is man usurping the power of God? Through Schwanthaler, Recolin argues that God has given man "beauty, illusion, and hope" in the world, and these are blessings. The truth is not. Schwanthaler treats his realization as one of ingratitude. He has wanted more than he possessed, and in the process of attaining it, he has thrown away the best part of human life—happiness in ignorance.

Each generation it seems must grapple in its own way with the paradox of dream and disappointment that X-ray vision carries. In 1933, it was American science fiction writer Edmond Hamilton's story "The Man with X-ray Eyes" published in the science fiction magazine *Wonder Stories*. David Winn, a young news reporter not unlike Clark Kent (Siegel and Shuster also read *Wonder Stories*), volunteers as the human test subject for a new series of eye drops that will give the user the power to see through walls. When asked about his reasons for wanting such power, he responds: "I would be the greatest reporter who ever lived! Don't you see what I mean? If I can look through walls and see what people are doing behind closed doors, I can get stories that no other reporter can get."[11] Once Winn receives this power, however, he discovers a world that is dishonest and unfair. He sees town leaders lying and business magnates cheating. He looks inside the prison, the hospital, and the slums, and the squalor, sickness, and death he witnesses is overwhelming. Winn's experiences result in him taking his own life: "he saw everything just as he wanted to and it was too much for him. God keep us blind in this world! Prevent us from the horror of doing what he did, of seeing—too well."[12] Winn's death reiterates the common 1930s message that X-ray vision and the knowledge that comes with it is beyond our capability. Each generation, however, asks the same question: What would we see if we could see all?

In 1963, the American pulp science fiction film *X: The Man with X-ray Eyes* took up the question. Starring Ray Milland and directed by Roger Corman, known for his low-budget horror films and highly influential on subsequent

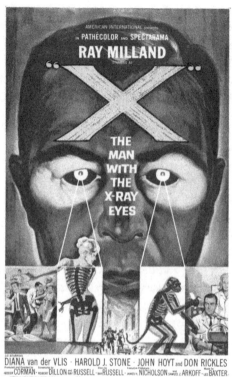

FIGURE 8 American pulp science fiction film *X: The Man with the X-ray Eyes* (1963) directed by Roger Corman. Poster by Reynold Brown. Public domain via Wikipedia Commons.

filmmakers including Francis Ford Coppola and Tim Burton, *X* tells the story of surgeon-scientist Dr. James Xavier who invents X, a liquid compound that gives him X-ray vision. Applied as eye drops, X has a cumulative effect; the more he takes, the more he can see. Lamenting that humans can see only ten percent of the wavelength of light, leaving them "blind to all but a tenth of the universe," Xavier imagines what he can do with his new vision: "In this hospital, there are people I can help. Help by seeing inside them, as if they were windows. By seeing their sicknesses with a clarity that would make X-rays a tool fit only for witchdoctors."[13] His friend Sam, an optometrist, warns Xavier that "only the gods see everything," to which Xavier replies: "My dear doctor, I'm closing in on the gods."[14]

Empowered but increasingly dependent on X, Xavier kills his assistant Brant when he attempts an intervention. Xavier goes on the run, hiding out at a carnival as Mentalo, a mystic seer. When he is discovered, he flees again with his manager, played by Don Rickles, and sets up as a gifted healer who can diagnose through sight. When Diane, Xavier's love interest, discovers him, the two flee to Las Vegas where Xavier uses his X-ray vision to win at blackjack. They plan to use the winnings to go to Mexico together, but when he is questioned by the casino manager, chaos ensues. In the melee, Xavier's light-blocking glasses are dislodged. At the sudden influx of light, Xavier screams and clutches at his eyes. The point-of-view shot shows viewers what he sees—a distorted room of prismatic skeletons.

Escaping from the casino and leading police on a high-speed chase into the desert, the final scene sees Xavier stumbling into a Christian revivalist tent meeting. When asked if he wants to be saved, Xavier slowly looks up at the camera, revealing that his eyes have turned completely black, and answers: "Saved? No. I've come to tell you what I see. There are great darknesses, farther than time itself. And beyond the darkness, a light that glows and changes. And in the center of the universe, the eye that sees us all."[15] The preacher yells that Xavier sees sin and the Devil, but God has given him the solution in Matthew 5:29: "If thine eye offends thee, pluck it out!"[16] Members of the congregation take up the chant: "Pluck it out! Pluck it out! Pluck it out! Pluck it out! Pluck it out!"[17] As the chanting continues, Xavier thrusts his hands to his eyes, his fingers curled inward, and lowers his head. When he raises his head up a few seconds later, his black eyes have been gouged out, replaced with empty red sockets. With this final act, the film ends.

If light is the real horror in *X: The Man with the X-ray Eyes*, then so too are the things it stands for: knowledge and insight. Like Schwanthaler and Winn before him, Xavier finds himself unable to cope with what he sees and with what he knows. More than once, Xavier expresses his longing for darkness, for the ability to shut his eyes and see nothing, to know nothing. But X has a cumulative effect. The more he takes, the more powerful his vision becomes, until he sees into a space beyond—the knowledge of which forces him to tear out his eyes.

To represent Xavier's X-ray vision, filmmakers used Spectarama, a new photographic technique that creates colorful but distorted prismatic effects. Developed in 1960 by Jon Howard, Spectarama gave the film colorful special effects that expand, contract, and spin onscreen. It has all the look and feel of an LSD-induced trip. American horror author Stephen King, whose work was also influenced by Corman's films, claims there was an additional line of dialogue that was cut because it was too horrific. In this alleged alternate ending, after gouging his eyes out, Xavier yells "I can still see!" In a 2017 interview, Corman denied there ever was such an ending, but added: "Now it's interesting, Stephen King saw the picture and wrote a different ending, and I thought, 'His ending is better than mine.'"[18] In the sixty years since the film's release, several directors, including Burton, have expressed interest in remaking it, though none have yet to do so.

The potential eye-gouging nightmare of X-ray vision does not deter our desire to experience the world through it. In 1964, the year after *X: The Man With X-ray Eyes* premiered, Harold N. Braunhut released his popular optical illusion glasses under the name X-Ray Specs. With their distinctive black-and-white swirled lenses, the X-ray glasses were advertised in the back pages of comic books with ads that highlighted their ability to "see bones thru skin" or "See living skeletons with these mystery X-ray glasses." The illusion relies on a polarizing effect created by a feather placed between the layers of each lens. The effect gives objects the look of a transparent outline with a solid center.

In 1999, the James Bond franchise released *The World is Not Enough* which prominently featured 007 wearing X-ray glasses. Distinguished as blue-tinted spectacles, Bond uses the glasses to see the concealed weapons, as well as the lingerie, of women around him. X-ray glasses are not nearly as popular today as they were in the 1960s or 1970s. They've been replaced by mobile phone apps that claim to turn one's phone into an X-ray camera.

These apps are free and obviously fake. Several of them state upfront that they are prank apps, but this does not stop people from believing that they are real: "I thought I broke my toe and so I downloaded this app and it does nothing so it wasted my time please do not download this app to check to see if something is broken because this app won't show you!! 😠😠😠😠."[19] And another: "This is stupid! I hit my middle finger really hard on the ground and wanted to see if the bone was injured at all. This app was just a white screen, only detecting my TV. I hate this app. I am not happy with the results. Try to make an app that ACTUALLY WORKS."[20] And these are just two reviews from hundreds that express similar frustrations, but why are they so angry? X-ray camera apps, like X-ray glasses before them, offer to democratize a technology and a power that belongs to the elite (doctors and radiologists) or the elect (superheroes). When the apps, like the glasses, are revealed to be nothing more than illusions, the anger of users is still very real. Even though our phones are powerful objects capable of emitting radiofrequency radiation (used to send signals), it's probably for the best that they cannot emit the ionizing radiation needed to create real X-rays.

Roentgen's discovery unlocked a way of knowing, measuring, mapping, and seeing the world that was previously unavailable to us. Like Dr. Xavier, however, we are constantly striving to see beyond the boundaries of our known world. All celestial bodies, from the planets to the stars, emit X-ray wavelengths to varying degrees, but because Earth's atmosphere absorbs most of these, the only way to study them is through X-ray telescopes and X-ray satellites. At NASA's Jet Propulsion Laboratory in Pasadena, California, scientists use NuSTAR, the Nuclear Spectroscopic Telescope Array launched in 2012, to detect high-energy X-ray light between 5 and 80 kiloelectron volts emitted by exploding stars, microflares on the sun, and the hot gases that surround black holes. Comparatively, NASA's Chandra, which launched on July 23, 1999, measures X-ray light energies in the lower spectrum between .01 and 10 kiloelectron volts. Together, NuStar and Chandra help scientists map the solar system and reveal its hidden workings. With these technologies, we have created the ability to see invisible light emanating from the depths of space—we have created X-ray vision on a cosmic level. By harnessing the power of X-rays, we are transcending the limits of our visible world.

4 EXPOSURE

"I don't have a Racist bone in my body!"
— PRESIDENT TRUMP, TWITTER, 2019

While X-ray vision remains elusive, X-rays do bifurcate our vision of the world, revealing glimpses of another world hidden beneath the one we readily see. With their discovery, X-rays proffered a radical new kind of intimacy and knowledge based on the belief that to see a thing is to know it—and the more we can see, the more we can know. Thus, the declaration "I see!" is a statement of understanding. X-rays expose new truths, but they also raise questions about the nature of knowledge. How do we *know* something or someone? And, what happens when X-rays reveal that our perception does not encompass the whole truth? In art and politics, X-rays and X-ray motifs capture the complex and troubled relationships between surface and depth, authenticity and superficiality, truth and lies. In a world where seeing is believing, can we ever trust what we see?

When radiology was still in its infancy, Dain Tasker, chief radiologist at Wiltshire Hospital in Los Angeles, began taking radiographs, or X-ray portraits. Often using himself as the subject, Tasker was drawn to the artistic possibilities that X-rays afforded. In his self-portrait, Tasker stands in profile, the outline of his glasses clearly visible atop an apparition of nasal cartilage. And while these images are interesting, they are not his most famous works. Drawn to the natural world, Tasker's most memorable and important work was done with flowers. In his floral radiographs, Tasker exposes the hidden structures inside orchids, lotuses, irises, fuchsias, tulips, birds of paradise, and lilies. Transparent and devoid of their usual striking colors, the flowers become beautifully uncanny, exposing a secret second self. Tasker's work gave viewers a new way to see, experience, and study the natural world without destroying it. His work even drew the attention of famed American photographer and environmentalist Ansel Adams, who printed Tasker's most famous image *X-ray of a Lily* (1930). Standing against a white background is a single calla lily. Under the X-ray's gaze, the white spathes that drape and sheath the spadix turn transparent, leaving the erect spadix exposed and on display. A haunting and erotic image, it entices us to look closer, to see what was withheld previously from our gaze.

From their origins, X-rays have been about voyeurism. The X-ray of Anna Bertha's hand wasn't just sensational; it was sexual. It gave viewers an intimate glimpse inside her body. Today, X-ray artists, like UK-based photographer

Nick Veasey, use X-rays to play with themes of surface and depth. In *X-Ray Voyeurism* (2014), Veasey created X-ray portraits of people going about their day, giving viewers the chance to stare unreservedly and to see what they carried inside their pockets and bags and bodies. One portrait is of an older woman pulling a suitcase behind her. Inside her body, we see an artificial hip, but inside her suitcase, we see a ball of yarn, a pair of knitting needles, and a spiked gimp mask staring back at us. The juxtaposition of the woman's body and bag speak to our own assumptions and voyeuristic desires. Other figures in this series include an exotic dancer, a corporate executive, and a punk rocker. With each, Veasey shows us something we expect and something we do not. In a corresponding series titled *Empty*, Veasey X-rayed sex dolls and sex toys: "Normally an X-ray reveals something hidden, but with this project I was trying to concentrate on things in life that flatter to deceive, don't live up to expectations, are vacuous."[1] Veasey uses the X-ray to show the emptiness of those objects to which people turn, voids to fill and be filled by. Like Tasker with his flowers, Veasey uses the X-ray medium to expose what is withheld, from secret pleasures to secret longings.

To art, the X-ray offered a new way of seeing and a new way of assessing. Today, whether they are preparing exhibitions, researching their collections, conserving works, or authenticating pieces, curators and art conservation experts regularly X-ray works of art to understand them better. A century ago, however, this idea was new and experimental and met with skepticism. In 1925, contemporaneous with Dain Tasker, Alan Burroughs, then the curator of paintings at the Minneapolis Art Institute, began using X-rays as an exploratory tool to study a painting's construction. With X-ray images, also known as X-radiographs, Burroughs claimed that one could extract hidden knowledge from inside the painting. X-rays made it possible to see an artist's process, to determine if different hands had worked on a piece, and to expose a fake or a forgery.

From 1925 to 1928, Burroughs undertook a large-scale examination of paintings at museums and archives across Europe using a portable X-ray machine. Burroughs found that the X-ray could not be fooled the way a human eye might be by repairs or retouching. An X-ray could more readily illuminate the work of different artists on the same painting by showing differences in brushwork, the application of paint, even the thickness of paint, all of which could be used as evidence of specific artists' work. Burroughs found that "by enabling the critic to become more intimate with the insides of pictures, the first thoughts of artists and any struggles inherent in the artistic process, the X-rays may guide the critic to new critical truths."[2]

Burroughs was not the first person to X-ray art, but he was the first trained curator and art historian to do so. In his ground-breaking book *Art Criticism from a Laboratory* (1938), Burroughs argues that shadowgraphs (his term for the images he created) could show not only new truths of a work, but it could reveal the workmanship and evidence of the artist's human touch. In discussing Leonardo da Vinci's *Virgin of the Rocks* which hangs in the National Gallery in London (an earlier version hangs in the Louvre), Burroughs reveals fingerprints in the paint that are only visible through the X-rays: "The fingerprints or hand-prints which show in the shadowgraph . . . must have been made in the pigment when soft, since they would not be recorded by the rays if they were made in varnish, which is not dense."[3] Preserved in the pigment but invisible to the naked eye, these prints belonging to an assistant or possibly da Vinci himself capture the moment of creation.

By their nature, X-rays are intimate, and Burroughs's shadowgraphs proffered a new and radical intimacy with art and artists. In his own words: "the X-ray, penetrating to the skeletons of pictures, adds to the subject matter of criticism the underpaint and preparatory workmanship . . . one may rely on X-ray shadowgraphs to show the development of an idea and the actual workmanship by which preliminary intention is transformed."[4] The X-ray offers to peel back layers of time, bifurcating our view to past and present, a work complete and a work in progress, decision and repentance.

Pentimenti, from the Italian *pentirsi* meaning to repent, are changes an artist makes in a painting and then covers up. These can be small changes, such as the movement of a hand, or larger reworkings. X-rays help us see and study *pentimenti*, offering viewers a glimpse into an artist's decision-making process. For example, many of Picasso's works from his blue period reveal different paintings underneath—not surprising as Picasso was broke during this period. X-rays of his 1902 painting *La Miséreuse Accroupie*, or *The Crouching Beggar*, reveal a landscape painting. Underneath *The Old Guitarist*, his famous 1903 painting of an old man stooped over playing guitar, is the apparition of an old woman, a young mother with her child, and a cow.

Finding *pentimenti* under a work one knows well can also be unsettling. Thomas Gainsborough's *The Blue Boy* (1770) is a full-length oil on canvas portrait of a young boy in a seventeenth-century blue suit of clothes set against a rather dark background. X-rays taken in 1939, 1994, and 2018 to 2019 reveal that the painting began life very differently. The canvas on which the portrait was made was cut down from a larger piece and reused; previously, it held the image of an old man. Originally sitting at the boy's feet was also a fluffy white dog, probably an English water spaniel. This singular *pentimento*, however, has been entombed inside a pile of rocks in the final portrait. Visible only on the X-ray, the ghostly companion waits patiently at the boy's feet.

It's unclear why Gainsborough regretted the dog and painted over it; perhaps he feared the dog would pull focus from the boy. No one knew the dog was there until the painting was X-rayed for the second time in 1994. Upon seeing the images, Shelley Bennet, the then-curator of British and European art at the Huntington Art Gallery where the portrait hangs, exclaimed: "I thought I knew these paintings, but I didn't know them."[5] The X-rays exposed the painting's long-held secrets, revealing the painting and the painter's creative process in new ways. When one visits Gainsborough's *The Blue Boy* today, its X-rays are displayed alongside it, revealing the dog underneath the pile of rocks. This doubling gives viewers the illusion of X-ray vision; we can see the finished work and simultaneously what lies beneath it.

X-rays have created a new field of knowledge by which art historians, conservators, and viewers can experience a work in all its layered complexities, revisions, erasures, miseries, and triumphs. From his expeditions to museums across Europe and the United States, Burroughs made over 4000 X-radiographs. In the process, he created a new kind of archive, one that granted the viewer a closer look at the process by which works were created and could assist in authenticating works and exposing fakes and forgeries. Now at the Fogg Art Museum at Harvard, the Alan Burroughs Collection of X-Radiographs houses 8000 X-radiographs made from approximately 5000 works of art from around the world. Much of the Alan Burroughs Collection has been digitized and is available to view online.

We like to look at X-rays of famous objects because we equate insight with intimacy. We think that by knowing the depths of a thing, or a person, we possess a secret knowledge and power over them. This is why celebrity X-rays are strange and funny things. From Muhammad Ali's jaw and Albert Einstein's skull to Marilyn Monroe's chest, celebrity X-rays reveal that they are human, just like us, but that is not why we are drawn to them. Marilyn Monroe's chest X-rays, taken in 1954 at Cedars of Lebanon Hospital in Florida where the actress underwent surgery, were sold in 2010 for $45,000 (approximately $63,300 in 2024). According to Darren Julien, owner of Julien's Auctions, the X-rays are "the ultimate look into the legend."[6] After all, what could be more personal than to see inside another individual?

In 2011, Kim Kardashian had her butt X-rayed to prove to her sisters (and the world) that she did not have implants—that her assets were authentic. Kardashian's X-rays were met with skepticism, but she and others pointed to them as proof that there were no implants, proof of her authenticity. While X-rays can pick up solid opaque objects within the body, such as silicone implants, they cannot detect fat transfers, that is when fat is taken from one part of the body and injected into another part. X-rays cannot prove without a doubt that Kim Kardashian has not undergone cosmetic *pentimenti*.

X-rays of rulers, politicians, and presidents have always drawn a big crowd. In 1896, the Duke and Duchess of York, later known as King George V and Queen Mary (grandparents to Queen Elizabeth II), were among the first royals to have their X-rays taken. In 2011, dental X-rays from the 1960s of Queen Elizabeth II and her father King George VI were pulled from the auction block after the royal family requested their removal, deeming the images too intimate. In the United States, visitors to the Ronald Reagan Museum in Simi Valley, California can see the chest X-rays taken after Reagan was shot in 1981 by John Hinckley Jr. They can also see the bullet that was lodged in Reagan's chest, half an inch from his heart, a bullet that could have changed history had it not been for X-rays. When Reagan collapsed on March 30, 1981 outside a Washington DC hotel as he walked to his motorcade, it was unclear that he had been shot. Reagan's own physician thought the President might be having a heart attack, but when doctors X-rayed him at the hospital, they saw the bullet. The following surgery to extract it saved Reagan's life.

Another president who might have been saved by the X-ray—but ultimately wasn't—was the 25th American President William McKinley, who was shot twice on September 6, 1901. McKinley survived the initial shooting, and while doctors were able to extract the first bullet, they could not locate the second bullet lodged in his stomach. McKinley had been attending the Pan-American Exposition in Buffalo, New York, where an X-ray machine was on display, but it was never used on McKinley, with some reports suggesting doctors were wary of harmful side effects. Receiving word of the assassination attempt, Thomas Edison sent one of his own portable X-ray machines from Menlo Park in New Jersey, but it too was never used (accounts differ as to why). Instead, unable to locate the bullet, doctors sutured McKinley's stomach closed and hoped for the best. After several days and appearing to be on the pathway to recovery, McKinley developed gangrene and died on September 14, 1901. An autopsy revealed it was not the bullet that killed him, but the gangrene and sepsis which had set in, most likely the product of surgeons' earlier efforts to locate the bullet in McKinley's stomach. While an X-ray saved Reagan and might have helped to save McKinley, it couldn't save Kennedy.

After his assassination in Dallas, Texas on November 22, 1963, X-rays of Kennedy's skull were taken as part of the autopsy investigation. Since then, they have been at the center of countless conspiracy theories and the four US government investigations that spawned them: the Warren Commission (WC) Report in 1964, the Clark Panel Report in 1968, the Rockefeller Commission in 1975, and the US House Select Committee on Assassinations (HSCA) in 1978. When the HSCA published its report in 1978, they included enhanced images of the X-rays that revealed notable differences from the original X-rays. With each investigation and report, the X-rays, autopsy photographs, and notes have been re-examined and re-interpreted by reputed pathologists and radiologists, but each report has only deepened the theories surrounding Kennedy's death. While I do not have the space in this book to examine the details of each report's interpretation of the X-rays and autopsy notes, I want to highlight the centrality of Kennedy's cranial X-rays and the conspiracy theories they have generated.

Of note are the differences in entry point location (the HSCA report moves the entry point up about 10 cm on the posterior of the skull, compared to the WC report), the exact damage done to Kennedy's skull, and the claims that there was a mysterious 6.5 mm metallic fragment embedded in Kennedy's skull or brain, but which was not reported in the original autopsy notes. Kennedy's brain, which was initially preserved, disappeared from the National Archives in 1966 along with other autopsy materials, generating an entirely different set of conspiracy theories about Kennedy's health and assassination. Since the release of the WC report, theorists have claimed that the original X-ray images were altered (possibly through double exposures) to obfuscate whether Kennedy was shot from the front or behind, the precise trajectory, the angle of the bullet, how many bullets hit Kennedy (the single bullet theory or "magic bullet" theory), and the type of bullets used (hollow point bullets, which can fragment on impact, or full metal jacket bullets, which do not fragment) with the claim that more than one type of bullet would suggest more than one shooter. Wielded by historians and conspiracy theorists, the X-rays and the autopsy reports have served paradoxically as evidence of the truth *and* evidence of a cover up. Ultimately, the contradictory readings of the X-rays have only deepened the debates and intensified the uncertainties surrounding Kennedy's assassination, leaving the truth ever more elusive.

The quest for truth finds an intriguing parallel in the rich history of political art, where the use of X-rays as metaphors for deceit and corruption dates back to 1896. Like X-rays, political cartoons have the power to expose the truth. This connection has contemporary relevance in the wake of President Trump. On July 16, 2019, in response to criticism of his tweets attacking minority Democratic congresswomen, Trump tweeted, "Those tweets were NOT Racist. I don't have

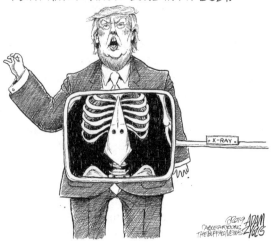

FIGURE 9 Editorial Cartoon by Adam Zyglis, 2019. Published originally in *The Buffalo News*. © Adam Zyglis. Courtesy of Cagle Cartoons.

a Racist bone in my body!"[7] Adam Zyglis, a Pulitzer Prize winning editorial cartoonist with *The Buffalo News*, captured the moment in a cartoon where Trump repeats his tweet as he stands behind an X-ray fluoroscope screen that reveals Trump's spine is in reality a Klu Klux Klan hood. As a visual metaphor, the X-ray works like a lie detector, exposing the truth of Trump—white supremacy is at his core. The cartoon underscores the enduring power of scrutiny and the search for truth symbolized by the X-ray.

Zyglis's cartoon was just one of several editorial and satirical responses to Trump's claim. *New York Magazine*'s *Intelligencer* ran an article with the headline "Contrary to Claims, X-ray Reveals that Trump has *Very* Racist Right Tibia" and an X-ray image of a tibia with "#NotMyAriel" stamped on it, a reference to the casting of Halle Bailey as Ariel in Disney's 2023 live-action *The Little Mermaid*. During his 2016 campaign, when Trump claimed that his bone spurs kept him from enlisting during the Vietnam War, a meme was born. The meme? An X-ray of a chicken's foot with the caption "Donald Trump's 'Bone Spur' X-ray Finally Released." In 2019, after Trump disparaged the late Senator John McCain, former Nebraska Senator and Navy Seal Bob Kerrey, who lost part of his right leg in Vietnam, called for Trump to show the nation X-rays of his feet, "because you don't grow out of bone spurs."[8] An X-ray would silence the bone spur doubters once and for all, Kerrey suggested. Despite the call for evidence, Trump has yet to produce any such X-ray.

The visual nature of political art allows for artists to communicate subversive messages directly to the public and empower people to acts of political resistance. X-rays in political art symbolize the desire to strip away the superficial layers of political rhetoric to reveal the hidden inner workings. In the 1930s, German visual artist John Heartfield (1891–1968) was best known for his radical anti-Nazi photomontages that deployed photography and Nazi imagery in subversive forms, such as a swastika made from bloody battle axes, or the dove of peace speared on a bayonet. Published in the communist magazine *Arbeiter-Illustrierte-Zeitung* (*AIZ*) on July 17, 1932, Heartfield's *Adolf der Übermensch*, or *Adolf the Superman*, is a photomontage that places a photograph of Adolf Hitler's head, his face frozen mid speech, atop a chest X-ray wherein Hitler's throat and stomach are visibly full of gold coins. The caption reads "Adolf, der Übermensch: Schluckt Gold und redet Blech" or "Adolf, the Superman: Swallows Gold and spouts Tin," to show the hypocrisy of Hitler's presenting himself as a working man when he was financially supported by wealthy German industrialists. Heartfield uses the X-ray to look beyond the façade of Hitler's rhetoric and speech-making and expose his corruption and greed. Heartfield's brother organized the printing and posting of hundreds of copies of *Adolf der Übermensch* throughout the streets of Berlin as a public warning and an act of political resistance.

In 1942, American artist B.F. Long produced the Axis Series, a series of political cartoons printed on postcards. The series featured X-ray cartoons of the insides of enemies' brains with the option to choose between Hitler, Mussolini, or Hirohito. Inside Hitler's brain, for example, are the objects that occupy his thoughts, such as a gun, a noose, a baby, a rat, a swastika armband, a leg with the word Liberty on it chained to an 8-lb weight, a globe, and a Nazi powder keg. The back of the postcard lists what these objects symbolize: "POWDER KEG—Has tried to blow civilization to pieces. BABY—Wants more babies for cannon fodder. GUN—

Has a gun at every head in Europe," and so on. Despite the differences between the artistic styles of Long, Heartfield, and Zyglis, collectively they use the X-rays for the same purpose: to expose a truth.

Exposure compels us to confront unsettling truths that we may prefer to avoid. At the Woodson Research Center at Rice University in Houston, Texas, the Dick Hedges World War II Memorabilia Collection is a small archive. Dixon "Dick" Hedges was a member of the Military Intelligence Center during World War II. He was among those responsible for transporting high-ranking Nazi officers to Nuremberg for the post-war trials. During his trips to Europe, Hedges kept a diary and collected Nazi memorabilia, including a set of X-rays taken of Hitler. Seeking medical attention for a perforated eardrum sustained during the July 20 plot, when German military leaders attempted to assassinate him, Hitler had a series of X-rays taken between September and October 1944 under the care of his personal physician Prof Dr. Theo Morrell. After Hitler's death, the Military Intelligence Service, to which Dick Hedges belonged, took Hitler's medical files and detained Morrell, who helped intelligence agents read the X-rays and write a report titled "Hitler As Seen By His Doctors." A copy of this report is in Hedges's collection, as well as the National Library of Medicine in Washington DC. The report indicates that some of the information contained within it was produced from Morrell's memory along with the files and records obtained by military intelligence in the aftermath of Hitler's death and the end of the war.

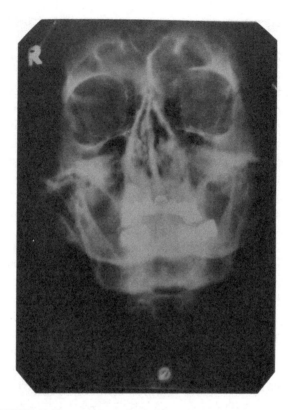

FIGURE 10 X-ray of Hitler's Skull, Dick Hedges WWII Memorabilia Collection, 1944-1945. Courtesy of the Woodson Research Center, Fondren Library, Rice University.

In total, there are five X-rays taken from three viewpoints: "the frontal sinus (nose-forehead position), the sphenoidal sinuses (mouth-chin position), and the maxillary, ethmoidal and frontal sinuses (chin-noise position)."[9] From the X-rays, it's easy to see that Hitler was in poor health. His nasal cavity and sinuses show signs of damage along with a pronounced leftward curve in his septum. The most disturbing bit, however, are his teeth. Hitler was known for having bad teeth, including chipped teeth, loose teeth, and missing crowns, that required serious dental reconstruction. The X-rays show that by October 1944, he retained only five of his original teeth. The rest of his mouth glows with a distinctive and complex combination of gold crowns, porcelain veneers, and a permanently affixed dental bridge that spans the roof of his mouth. Since May 1945, rumors persisted that Hitler survived the war and escaped Germany, but in 2017, his X-rays would be key to proving that he did not.

Hitler left orders that his body be burned after his death on April 30, 1945. When Soviet forces reached the Führerbunker on May 2, 1945, they found among the charred remains of several bodies jaw fragments containing gold teeth, dental prostheses, and bridgework. Believing the remains to be Hitler's, Soviet officers assigned 25-year-old Elena Rzhevskaya, a Russian Jew working as a translator for the Soviet army, to carry the jaw fragments and teeth to Berlin. She was deemed the most reliable to keep the remains secure and secret. Reaching Berlin, Soviet forces were able to capture Fritz Echtmann, the dental technician who had made Hitler's bridgework, and Käthe Heusermann, a dental assistant. Interrogated by Soviets with the help of Elena Rzhevskaya, Echtmann and Heusermann drew sketches and described in detail the dentistry and bridgework Hitler had received. Their information matched the remains.

In the first days of May 1945, Soviet leader Joseph Stalin knew Hitler was dead, but he suppressed the information, reluctant for America and Britain to know that Hitler had died. Stalin made Hitler's death and the discovery of Hitler's remains a state secret; disclosure carried a 15-year-sentence to the gulag prison camp. To guarantee their silence, Käthe Heusermann and Fritz Echtmann were imprisoned until after Stalin's death in 1954. Elena Rzhevskaya, who had carried and helped identify Hitler's remains, also kept her experiences a secret until after Stalin's death. In 1954, she approached the Russian literary magazine *Znayma* with her memoirs, which the magazine published, but fearful of a potential backlash, they cut the section on Hitler's death and the identification of the teeth.

In December 2016 and May 2017, Russian President Vladimir Putin granted French journalist Jean-Christophe Brisard and Russian journalist Lana Parshina, along with French forensic pathologist Philippe Charlier, access to the Russian State Archives where the jaw fragments and teeth believed to belong to Hitler have been kept in secret since 1945. In their book *The Death of Hitler: The Final Word* (2018), Brisard and Parshina detail their and Charlier's forensic examination of the remains. Charlier determined that the jawbone, teeth, and dentures held in the Russian archives match those in Hitler's X-rays. They show evidence of being the right age and time period for Hitler's life and death; they show evidence of having been in a fire, as it was reported that Hitler's body was burned; and, they possess the same unique dental prostheses and bridgework shown in the X-rays.

The publication of Brisard and Parshina's book in 2018 coincided with the English translation of Rzhevskaya's memoir, *Memories of a Wartime Interpreter: From the Battle for Moscow to Hitler's Bunker*, which included the sections about her role as courier of Hitler's remains. In 2018, newspapers from America to Australia ran articles announcing that Hitler's teeth confirmed his death. Since 1945, rumors have persisted that Hitler escaped and survived. The X-rays matched to the remains prove that he did not.

When I learned that Hitler's X-rays still existed, I knew I needed to see them for myself. Sitting in the Woodson Research Center in Houston, Texas on a hot humid day in July, they arrived in the reading room in a gray archival box labeled "X-rays of Hitler's Head" and "RESTRICTED." Inside were the five X-rays, each one in its own protective plastic envelope. As I lifted each one out and arranged them on the table, I slipped my fingers beneath the plastic protectors. I had to touch them. In researching this book, I've seen and held a lot of X-rays: X-rays of men wounded in war; of children who've swallowed things; of TB patients;

even those of a friend who broke her ankle the summer I began writing this book. Holding the Hitler X-rays was different.

Produced on Kodak Safety-2 film, a cellulose-acetate X-ray film that is thicker than the type used today, the X-rays have weight to them, and their surface feels slick. Modern X-ray film feels tackier, like plastic; Hitler's X-rays feel almost metallic. Like old daguerreotypes, they are bordered by a silver-sheen edge, a few centimeters wide. Distinctly visible in the silver border are fingerprints.

Hitler's X-rays are haunting. They are disturbing and upsetting, the embodiment of evil. When Hitler's doctors examined these, no doubt they saw physical manifestations of pain and the evidence of pain that he experienced. That is what X-rays do after all, locate pain. When we examine these X-rays today, however, what are we looking for? We want answers, because we equate X-rays with exposure and the truth. These X-rays, however, hold no answers, at least not to the important questions. To see, hold, and touch these X-rays does not offer more insight into Hitler or the origins of his horrifying inhumanity. Instead, the only thing these X-rays expose is a truth we want to reject—that for all his atrocities, Hitler was undeniably human.

In the 1930s, Superman, created by two sons of Jewish families, restored public trust in X-rays by aligning X-ray vision with truth and justice, steeping the narrative of X-rays in their power to expose evil and fight injustice. So frequently the story of X-rays is about what they reveal, that we never consider the power of X-rays to cover up or how concealment can be its own act of political resistance.

Starting as early as the 1940s, underground music bootleggers in the USSR repurposed X-ray film by turning it into music. At the time, Soviet music, art, and culture were controlled by the state, which believed that cultural productions and expressions must be made in service to the state and tightly controlled by censors. Western music and culture were forbidden, but this didn't stop its being smuggled into the country through port cities like St. Petersburg. At the same time, the film X-rays were made on was combustible and highly flammable, so it was routine for hospitals to discard used X-ray films with some regularity. Music bootleggers salvaged it because X-ray film is a type of vinyl plastic. Using homemade record lathes, they could record forbidden Western music directly onto the X-rays. The favored genres included rock & roll, blues, and jazz and music by Elvis Presley, The Beatles, the Rolling Stones, and Ella Fitzgerald.

Exchanged on the black market, the thin X-ray-film records could be stashed up coat sleeves or tucked under a shirt at a moment's notice. These X-ray records became symbols of resistance against censorship and oppression. Sometimes called "ribs" or "bone music," these X-rays, records of the physical pains of Soviet people, became weapons in an invisible war instigated by Soviet censors and played out over the invisible airwaves of radio. Bone music became emblematic both of people's pain and their joy.

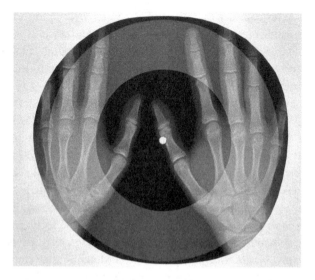

FIGURE 11 "Ribs" or "bone music" created by underground music bootleggers in the Soviet Union. This X-ray record features "Devil in Her Heart" (1963) by The Beatles. Author's photograph.

Many of these records survive and can be purchased in Eastern Europe, Russia, or online. I purchased two records from a large collection online, receiving an X-ray of two hands on which was recorded The Beatles' "Devil in Her Heart" (1963) and an X-ray of the upper vertebrae and base of the skull on which is recorded The Beatles' "Run for Your Life" (1965). The band and song titles have been etched in cursive into the blank space surrounding the play hole. Both songs are about betrayal, fitting since this music was once forbidden. When they arrived, the X-rays were inside thin paper sleeves reused from traditional vinyl records, further accentuating their identity not as X-ray images but as sound recordings. I asked an audiophile friend to help me play them, to see if their sound had been preserved; but after several attempts on multiple machines, we could only produce static. The thinness of the vinyl film meant that X-ray recordings could be played only a limited number of times before they deteriorated, like a built-in self-destruct feature, appropriate since making, selling, or buying forbidden music carried harsh, sometimes fatal, punishments. Holding these X-rays is a different experience than holding others because they expose the resilience and strength of people, not their weakness. While X-ray vision may belong only to imagined superheroes, X-ray motifs in art and politics are about democratizing the power of X-rays to expose the complex truths and lies that make up our world.

5 FOREIGN BODIES

"That punk pulled a Glock 7 on me. You know what that is? It's a porcelain gun, made in Germany. Doesn't show up on your airport X-ray machines"
— **JOHN MCCLANE, *DIE HARD 2: DIE HARDER***

A foreign body does not belong. In medicine, a foreign body is an object originating outside the body but which has gotten inside, either by accident or with intent, and must be removed. Regardless of size or material, everything in the body that does not belong is diagnosed as a *foreign body*. If we look at synonyms for foreign body, though, we get words like impurity, pollutant, stranger, alien, and outsider. X-rays expose what does not fit—the foreign body—which is why today, X-rays are synonymous with security, especially border security, and those borders are both personal and political.

Philadelphia is home to one of the most engrossing museums in America. The Mütter Museum, located at The

College of Physicians of Philadelphia, is famous for its vast collections of human organs, body parts, and pathological oddities. One can explore the history of human anatomy through permanent exhibits of human bones, organs, and diseased tissues preserved in formaldehyde. The museum houses a life-size plaster cast of Chang and Eng Bunker, famous conjoined twins, and the Hyrtl Skull Collection comprised of 139 human skulls collected by Viennese anatomist Josef Hyrtl (1810–1894). Also among the permanent collection is the foreign bodies collection of Dr. Chevalier Jackson (1865–1958) containing "2,374 inhaled or swallowed foreign bodies that Dr. Jackson extracted from patients' throats, esophaguses, and lungs during his almost 75-year-long career…. More than 80% of the patients were under 15 years old."[1] Now lauded as the father of endoscopy, Jackson, a laryngologist, developed his own original tools and techniques for removing objects from the throats and stomachs of patients, many of whom were small children or infants. Along with patient notes and the X-ray images that guided his hands, Jackson kept every single foreign body removed, including a quarter he removed from a child's throat, even after the child's father demanded it back. By themselves and out of context, the objects in the exhibit, from buttons and coins to toy jacks and even a small battleship, seem somewhat benign. It's not hard to imagine a small child swallowing any of these things, but looking at them evokes feelings of amazement and wonder, not fear. Fear comes from seeing the objects in situ on the X-rays.

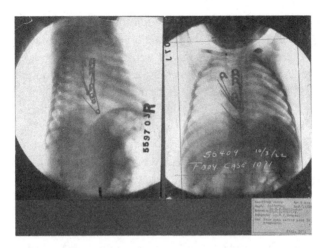

FIGURE 12 X-ray image from Chevalier Jackson's Case #1071. The four large open safety pins were wrapped in wool and allegedly fed to the nine-month-old baby by a sibling. Historical Medical Photographs-Chevalier Jackson skiagraphs, Esophagus Book II. Courtesy of the Historical Medical Library of the College of Physicians of Philadelphia.

Perhaps the most terrifying X-rays are those belonging to a nine-month-old infant. And the foreign body? A set of four large open safety pins, the kind used in the days before disposable diapers, threaded together at their hinges, and wrapped in a piece of fabric. Jackson's collection includes lots of safety pins of all sizes. When parents of previous generations pinned diapers or clothing on a child, they might momentarily hold the safety pin in their mouth. Children, especially babies, imitate their parents. When some children got hold of a safety pin, they naturally put it into their mouths and, if not stopped in time, swallowed it. In his autobiography, *The Life of Chevalier Jackson* (1938), Jackson reflects on this case, known as fbdy #1071, as his most difficult. One look at the X-ray shows why—this child's life was in Jackson's hands.

In her remarkable book *Swallow: Foreign Objects, Their Ingestion, Inspiration, and the Curious Doctor Who Extracted Them*, Mary Cappello writes: "the four pins, splayed, fully open, and pointing upward, appear to dwarf the baby's ribs in the X-ray, and the image is nearly overwhelming as a representation of *that which does not belong*, as a record of an uncanny disconnect between a body's interior and a piece of the world trapped therein."[2] At nine months old, the diameter of a child's esophagus is approximately 8 mm, about the size of a standard drinking straw. Working in a space that small, Jackson's task seems impossible. He had first to untangle the pins and close them. He then placed the two lower pins into the stomach to be passed through the child's gastrointestinal system, which they were, and extracted the upper two pins from the child's esophagus. The child survived and to all accounts recovered and led a normal life. Although not known for certain, it's believed that the child's four-year-old sibling fed the pins to him. For Jackson, X-rays images and X-ray fluoroscopes served as his eyes in the diagnoses and procedures to remove the foreign bodies from the throats and lungs of his tiniest patients. For the rest of his life, Jackson led awareness campaigns to educate families about the dangers that common household objects presented to children.

Obviously, it isn't just children who ingest things they shouldn't. Pets are notorious for gobbling up the things that comprise our daily lives—hair ties, jewelry, socks, golf balls, action figures—and often we're completely ignorant until we find a GI Joe in the litter box. Every year since 2006, *Veterinary Practice News* has held a "They Ate What?!" X-ray Contest on their website where veterinarians from around the world are invited to submit and vote on the wildest animal X-rays. Looking through the X-rays from the 2021 and 2022 contests, we find lots of children's toys, wedding rings, a nickel, and even a spoon. The more unusual objects include 169 small rocks (inside one dog), pieces of a turtle's shell, a spatula, two rubber ducks, eight pounds (yes, 8 lbs.) of hair ties, a 15-inch metal skewer complete with onion and meat chunks, and even a rubber chicken. My personal favorite was the dog that cannibalized a figurine of a dog. On the X-ray, the toy dog's placid eyes look out from between the real dog's ribs, a tiny plastic prisoner.

Since the 1960s, the Food and Drug Administration (FDA) has approved the use of X-rays in scanning food products to improve food safety, and on its website, the FDA suggests that irradiating food "improves the safety and extends the shelf life of foods by reducing or eliminating microorganisms and insects," comparing the practice to pasteurizing milk or canning vegetables.[3] Even NASA astronauts "eat meat that has been sterilized by irradiation to avoid getting foodborne illnesses when they fly in space."[4] That makes sense—space would be the worst place to have food poisoning. But when one asks people about X-raying food, most people (or at least, most Americans) will think of Halloween candy. In 2015, *Vice Magazine* ran the controversial headline, "Stop X-raying Your Kid's Halloween Candy." The accompanying article was in response to the annual tradition of American parents X-raying their kids' Halloween candy and featured an interview with Dr. Joel Best, a professor of sociology and criminal justice at the University of Delaware and "the leading expert on everything that maniacs are allegedly putting in your kids' candy."[5]

The earliest cases that Best documents as sources giving rise to the urban legend of poisoned Halloween candy are from the 1970s, notably the deaths of five-year-old Kevin Totson in Detroit, Michigan, who died on November 6, 1970 from candy allegedly laced with heroin, and eight-year-old Timothy O'Bryan in Pasadena, Texas, who died on Halloween 1974 after eating a Pixie Stix laced with cyanide. Later, it was revealed that Totson "had found the heroin in a relative's home."[6] Timothy O'Bryan, however, was killed with poisoned Halloween candy deliberately given to him by his father. Ronald Clark O'Bryan, who became known as 'The Candy Man,' 'The Trick-or-Treat Murderer,' and 'The Man Who Killed Halloween,' had a $20,000 life insurance policy on his son and had given Timothy and four other children the deadly candy. Timothy died one hour after eating the Pixie Stix, which he had complained tasted bitter. The other four children, including Timothy's five-year-old sister, survived. Although Ronald Clark O'Bryan never confessed, he was found guilty of his son's murder and four attempted murders and executed in Texas in 1984. Nevertheless, the fear and the urban legend of poisoned Halloween candy lives on.

Fueled by public panic after the deaths of Totson and O'Bryan and the Chicago Tylenol Murders of 1982, where seven people died after being sold Tylenol that had been laced with potassium cyanide, the American tradition of X-raying Halloween candy began. On October 30, 1985, *The Los Angeles Times* ran an article announcing that Orange County hospitals would offer free radiographic screening of Halloween candy: "In the interest of a safe Halloween, Orange County area hospitals and medical centers are offering free X-ray inspections of treats to detect the presence of any metallic foreign objects."[7] Larry Walters, the assistant director of radiology at Hoag Memorial Hospital Presbyterian in Newport Beach, clarified: "X-rays can detect nails, pins, needles, razor blades," but "what's important to note is we cannot detect poison."[8] The article goes on to cite two cases of contaminated candy in 1982, but these cases could not be verified.

Since the 1980s, Best has followed reports of "Halloween sadism" and alleged poisonous candy received from strangers on Halloween. His findings show that these cases are repeatedly misattributed, such as Totson's, or are outright hoaxes. In a 2015 interview, Best called for the end of X-raying Halloween candy. The process is costly, Best argues, and offers false security as X-rays cannot detect poisonous substances, such as cyanide or heroin, in candy or food. Despite the evidence and urging of Best and other experts, the American public is not persuaded. The X-raying of Halloween candy continues with several hospitals across the US offering to X-ray candy each year.

Public panic cannot be blamed entirely for this ritual. Our confidence in X-rays has been built across the decades, and we've been habituated to equate X-rays with safety and security. In 1970, the same year as Kevin Totson's death, the first walk-through metal detectors were installed in the New Orleans International Airport. Prior to 1970, there were no mass screenings of airline passengers or their luggage. Three years later, on January 5, 1973 at LAX, the first cabinet X-ray machines designed to scan passengers' luggage were switched on. Why were these security measures introduced? Because between May 1961 and December 1972 in the US, there were 159 passenger aircraft hijackings, with 130 occurring in the four years between 1968 and 1972. Worldwide, there were 326.

It was in a July 1968 Senate hearing that Florida Senator George Smathers first proposed the use of metal detectors or cabinet X-ray machines in airports: "I see no reason why similar devices couldn't be installed at airport check-in gates to determine whether passengers are carrying guns or other weapons just prior to emplaning."[9] FAA director Najeeb Halaby had rejected the proposal, and Irving Ripp, the FAA representative at the hearing, dismissed Smathers's suggestion citing that such measures would have "a bad psychological effect on passengers" and "people would complain about invasion of privacy."[10] The very next year, 1969, there were 40 hijackings in the US. Eleven of those occurred in the first three weeks of January. The FAA changed their minds.

It was FAA policy until the late 1960s to comply with hijackers' demands in the belief that it reduced the risks to passengers, but the dramatic rise in hijackings demanded action. John Dailey, the FAA's chief psychologist, convinced the agency to implement a system of passenger profiling based on physical characteristics and behaviors. This type of security relies entirely on human behaviors and perceptions; it is subjective and flawed as prejudice, human error, and fatigue can lead to missed threats resulting in disasters. In the 1960s, profiling alone was not enough. X-rays, impartial and indefatigable, restored a sense of control and security. And despite the FAA's fears of unhappy customers and the rise in ticket prices to cover the additional costs, customer surveys showed that passengers did not seem to mind the increased security.

It's this history that lies behind the plot of the 1990 blockbuster film *Die Hard 2: Die Harder*. The premise of the film is pretty simple: terrorists use porcelain guns to bypass the X-ray machines and airport security at Washington Dulles. They take control of the airport and threaten to crash passenger planes until their demands are met. The quote from Bruce Willis's character, Detective Lieutenant John McClane, at the beginning of this chapter is one of the film's most famous lines—because everything about it is wrong.

Glock isn't made in Germany; it's made in Austria. Glock has never made a Glock 7. Porcelain guns are a myth (porcelain is too brittle and would shatter on discharge), and porcelain *does* show up on X-rays. None of this, however, stopped the brief hysteria that resulted when *Die Hard 2* hit American movie theaters on the Fourth of July 1990.

After the film's release, fear over a super gun gripped the American public. Rumors of KGB plastic guns, which could bypass metal detectors, had been around since the 1970s, increasing in volume in 1987 when Florida gun maker David Byron filed a patent for an all-plastic gun. The timing of *Die Hard 2* was such that American audiences were ready to believe in the existence of an "invisible," or X-ray-proof, gun. The X-ray machine, the embodiment of border security, had been breached. Only it hadn't, not really. The hysteria was intense but brief, dying down within a few weeks. What it revealed was how ingrained the idea of X-rays as synonymous with security, especially airport security, had become since 1973. So, it makes sense that after the hijacking of four American passenger planes on September 11, 2001, we turned to X-rays once again to re-establish control and security.

The introduction of cabinet X-ray machines in 1973 had gone relatively smoothly. The introduction of the passenger-scanning backscatter X-ray machines in 2009 did not. Unlike traditional X-rays, backscatter X-rays do not pass through an object. Rather, they are reflected back or bounced off an object to create an image of it. For passengers, these X-rays are capable of scanning through clothing and creating a detailed image of the human form beneath, earning them the nickname "the naked X-rays." Their introduction inspired several inventors to create X-ray-proof underwear, echoing the same fears over privacy that people in 1896 expressed. In addition to X-ray-proof underwear, which was woven with tungsten fibers in a fig leaf pattern and sold online, there were also undershirts that when exposed to the backscatter X-rays showed TSA screeners a copy of the Fourth Amendment against unreasonable searches and seizures. In 2010, many people's fears were realized when detailed scans of passengers' bodies were leaked online; this exposure led, in part, to the removal of the more invasive machines in 2013.

In its 2022 annual report, TSA revealed they scanned 763 million people and confiscated 6,542 firearms. TSA also released its top ten weirdest things for 2022, including a gun stuffed inside a raw chicken; disassembled parts of a gun in jars of peanut butter; a knife in a laptop; thousands of fentanyl candies; and, a cattle prod in a guitar case. Well, that last one I can understand—deplaning takes too long. In the annals of TSA lore, there are even weirder objects, such as human skulls, and more dangerous ones, including live hand grenades, proving that despite their risks, X-rays in airports have never been more important to our safety and security.

In the wake of the naked X-rays and growing fears over dangerous levels of exposure to ionizing radiation in daily life, *The New York Post* published an October 2015 article with the headline "NYPD has super-secret X-ray vans."

Picked up in subsequent publications including *The Atlantic* and *International Business Times*, journalists covered the mysterious mobile X-ray vans that the NYPD operate around New York City to scan…who knows? Cars, people, buildings? When pressed for information, then-police commissioner Bill Bratton responded, "I will not talk about anything at all about this—it falls into the range of security and counter-terrorism activity that we engage in."[11] Freedom of Information requests about the vans have been ignored. To this day, there has not been a full disclosure of where or how the New York Police Department (NYPD) utilize mobile X-ray vans within the city. Rather, the public have been asked to trust in the NYPD's lawful and safe use of such technologies. Certainly, X-rays are central to national and personal security, and despite their invasive and dangerous properties, they make us feel assured of that security, but that trust ends when consent is ignored.

X-rays can save us in many ways, but can they save us from ourselves? In 1977, the *American Journal of Surgery* coined the euphemism "social injury of the rectum" to describe injuries sustained from objects inserted into the rectum for sexual pleasure. Around the same time, the United States Consumer Product Safety Commission established the National Electronic Injury Surveillance System (NEISS), which for the past 45 years has maintained a database of consumer-product injuries that required a visit to a hospital emergency room.

The NEISS database is public and searchable. Anyone can access it and peruse all manner of injuries caused by almost anything and affecting any part of the body. With consumer products ranging from toys and household appliances to fireworks and gardening equipment, there are injuries as benign as splinters and as gruesome as amputation, crushing, and death. It is a fascinating read of human frailty and folly.

But I'm here for only one thing: a query of "foreign body" and "lower trunk." I set my search parameters at five years between 2017 to 2021. It yields over 40,000 matching items. I add the search term "rectum," and my results reduce to 609 cases. Between 2017 and 2021, 609 individuals received emergency care for a foreign-body injury to, or in, the rectum. It is actually quite a small number compared to the over 40,000 foreign-body injuries to the lower trunk, which includes everything from embedded fishhooks and lost belly-button rings to impaled fence posts, or the almost 443,000 ingested objects recorded in the same period. Most of the foreign bodies in my search results are lost anal plugs, dildos, and vibrators—remember folks: without a base, without a trace—but not all of them. These are just some of the more unusual foreign bodies recorded in the NEISS database as causing injury to or in the rectum:

Shower spigot
Fishing pole
Wooden broom handle
Lightbulb
Candle
Christmas ornament

Perfume bottle

Shampoo bottle

Deflated balloon

2 LB dumbbell

Baseball

Two Poker Chips

#8 pool ball

Golf ball

Small foam football

Frozen jump rope handle

Barbie Doll head

12-inch carrot

Apple wrapped in paper towels

The NEISS database does not include personal information beyond age, sex, and race, but it does include the intake notes, which reveal some of the fascinating stories behind these objects. For example, the 69-year-old man who came into the ER with the frozen jump rope handle and claimed, he "sat down on [a] rag with chemicals on it" and that his "buttocks started burning."[12] So, he "put water in jump rope handle, froze it & put in rectum."[13] I guess that's not entirely implausible. Some of the patients are forthright, like the 45-year-old man who arrived "with 2 poker chips up rectum because of bet."[14] No mention of whether he lost or won the bet. Others are less forthcoming: "41[-year-old man] was playing with a container of athlete's foot spray and accidentally it ended up in his rectum."[15] There are actually quite a few *accidents*. "A million-to-one shot, doc. Million-to-one," as Frank says on *Seinfeld* in season six, episode twenty-one, better known as the Assman episode.[16]

The youngest patients are two or three years old who come to the ER with crayons, pennies, and even toy sharks lodged inside, acts born out of curiosity and a testing of personal boundaries. The oldest patient on record is an 81-year-old man who claimed: "He was using a water bottle to scratch his anus when the plastic cap came off and went into his rectum."[17] I'll give him the benefit of a doubt on this one.

While not all foreign-body injuries require X-rays, many of them do. Patients have sometimes had these objects lodged inside their bodies for hours, days, and even weeks. The NEISS database does not include the X-ray images, but that's okay. In this case, I do not need to see it to believe it. What the database does offer is an intimate story of people's secrets, their hidden lives, their pleasure as well as their pain.

X-rays can reveal our eccentricities and even our fetishes in embarrassing ways, but they are also part of our self-discovery. We can experiment with our bodies knowing that, if need be, X-rays can save us from the consequences of our actions. Despite all our worries and resistance to X-rays, we need them. They are emergency responders. They restore order. We trust X-rays to tell us the truth, to hold us together, to show us what lies beneath. They make us, you x me, feel safe in ourselves and in the world.

6 YOU X ME

One of my earliest tangible memories is of getting a chest X-ray. I was six years old and hospitalized with pneumonia. I can remember the light in the room, the metal table under me, and the feel of a cold board pressed against my naked back. Later, I remember seeing the X-ray—*my* X-ray—hanging from a lightboard as the doctor explained to my parents what it meant. I asked if I was going to die. No, I wasn't, and I didn't, but the uncanny sensation of seeing my skeleton outside my body has followed me ever since.

In March 2020, lockdowns, quarantines, and fear gripped the world as the Covid-19 global pandemic spread. In that same month, Alijan Ozkiral, a graduate student in English at New York University, and Christian Krenek, a theater scholar and teacher, submitted their proposal to Unicode for the addition of a new emoji: an X-ray. It was a proposal they had begun in 2019, but in March 2020, the pair demonstrated the need for it, noting the requests on social media for an X-ray emoji and the high probability of its usage. I don't think they anticipated just how much we would need an X-ray emoji in the weeks and months to come. Approved in 2021, the X-ray emoji was released in September 2021 as part of Unicode 14.0. And what was the first X-ray emoji? A chest X-ray.

While I've been thinking about X-rays for many years, the Covid-19 global pandemic has given them new significance. Before more accurate and rapid testing for Covid was developed and made widely available, chest X-rays were used for diagnosis. I think it's important to note that in the first moments of our global crisis, we turned to X-rays—a light we cannot see—for answers.

ACKNOWLEDGMENTS

want to thank series editors Ian Bogost and Christopher Schaberg for the opportunity to write this book, and Haaris Naqvi for his patient support and guidance. I am honored to be part of the Object Lessons series.

I am so grateful for the friendship and feedback of fellow Object Lesson writer Harry Brown (*Golf Ball*), whose mentorship helped me find my way. Special thanks to Object Lessons writers Sheila Liming (*Office*), Anna Leahy (*Tumor*), and Robert Bennett (*Pill*) for sharing their work with me as I planned this book.

Many thanks to the librarians and archival staff at the British Library, the Wellcome Collection, the London School of Economics Library, the National Archive at Kew, the Huntington Library, and the Harry Ransom Center for their knowledge and assistance through the research and early writing stages of this project. Additional thanks to the fellowship programs at the Huntington Library and the Harry Ransom Center at the University of Texas at Austin, which supported my research.

I owe my biggest thanks to my friends: Lisa, whose X-rays of her broken tibia were a timely source of inspiration; Lucy A and Lucy C, for the brainstorming sessions over iced coffees; Robert, who always sees the light in the dark; Deepa, for making me smile; and Ryan and Betsy, for always being there, making me laugh, and pouring the champagne.

Lastly, I want to thank my family—Julie, Kim, Casey, Michele, Rosemary, Joseph, Erin, Ryan, Abigail, and Mia—with whom everything is possible.

NOTES

Chapter 1

1   Joshua Bennett, "X," in *The Sobbing School* (New York: Penguin, 2016), 68.

2   Vincent J. Cirillo, "The Spanish-American War and Military Radiology," *American Journal of Roentgenology* 174, no. 5 (2000): 1237. https://doi.org/10.2214/ajr.174.5.1741233

3   Photographic prints with clinical notes on reverse, early 20th century, X-rays of First World War wounds, Professor Thomas Renton Elliott collection, GC/42/19, Contemporary Medical Archives Center, Wellcome Collection, London.

4   "X-rays of First World War Wounds." Professor Thomas Renton Elliott Collection, Wellcome Collection.

5   Otto Glasser, *Wilhelm Roentgen and the Early History of the Roentgen Rays* (San Francisco: Norman Publishing, 1993), 203.

6   Ibid., 45.

7   Ibid., 205.

8   From photocopy of incomplete letter from Josephine Butler to Stanley Butler, 5 March 1896, Josephine Butler Letters Collection, TWL 6.2 Box 4, 3JBL/35/21, The Women's Library, London School of Economics Library, London.

9   Philip C. Goodman, "The New Light: Discovery and Introduction of the X-ray," *AJR* 165, (November 1995): 1044.

10   Letter from Eric Barrington to Sir Frank Lascelles, 7 April 1896, FO 800–Foreign Office, Private Offices: Various Ministers' and Officials' Papers, Fo 800/9–Germany Volume 3, Part 1, Folios 36-37, FO 800/9/10, The National Archive, Kew.

11   "C.M. Dally Dies A Martyr to Science," *The New York Times,* October 4, 1904, 16.

12   "Edison Fears Hidden Perils of the X-Rays," *New York World*, August 3, 1903, 1.

13   L.E. Etter, "Some historical data relating to the discovery of the Roentgen rays," *The American Journal of Roentgenology and Radium Therapy and Nuclear Medicine* 56 (1946): 220–231.

Chapter 2

1   Anon., "X-actly So!," *Electrical Review* 38 (April 17, 1896): 511.

2   George Griffith, "A Photograph of the Invisible," *Pearson's Magazine* 1, no. 1 (April 1896): 380.

3   Ibid., 380.

4   H.G. Wells, *The Invisible Man* (Peterborough: Broadview Press, 2018), 119.

5   Ibid., 47-9.

6   Ibid., 75-6.

7   Ibid., 78.

8 Originally published in French as "Ja pense, donc je suise," in Descartes's 1637 work *Discours de la Méthode Pour bien conduire sa raison, et chercher la vérité dans les sciences*, or *Discourse on the Method of Rightly Conducting One's Reason and of Seeking Truth in the Sciences*. The Latin version did not appear until 1644 in Descartes's *Principles of Philosophy*.

9 Barbara Johnson, *Persons and Things* (Cambridge: Harvard University Press, 2008), 51.

10 H.G. Wells, *The Invisible Man* (Peterborough: Broadview Press, 2018), 169.

11 "X-ray Skirts Break Up Home of Millionaire," *Oregon Daily Journal*, September 5, 1913, 1.

12 Worton David and Bert Lee, "In Your X-ray Gown" (London: Francis, Day and Hunter, 1913), 4.

13 "Posture Contests are Big Business," *Digest of Chiropractic Economics* 1, no. 1 (July 1958): 4.

Chapter 3

1 Harry Houdini, *Houdini exposes the tricks used by the Boston Medium 'Margery' to win the $2500 prize offered by the Scientific American: Also a complete exposure of Argamasilla the famous Spaniard who baffled noted Scientists of Europe and America, with his claim to X-ray vision* (New York: Adams Press Publisher, 1924), 33.

2 Ibid., 33.

3 Ibid., 36.

4 William Woolfolk, "The Man of Steel's Super Manhunt," *Superman #59* (New York: DC Comics, 1949).

5 Joel Shuster, Jerry Siegel, and Joanne Siegel, "Of Supermen and Kids with Dreams," interview by Tom Andrea, Geoffrey Blum, and Gary Coddington, *NEMO: The Classic Comics Library #2* (August 1983): 9.

6 Beatriz Colomina, *X-ray Architecture* (Zurich: Lars Müller Publishers, 2019), 147.

7 C. Henry Kempe, M.D., Frederic N. Silverman, M.D., Brandt F. Steele, M.D., et al., "The Battered Child Syndrome," *Journal of the American Medical Association*, 181.1 (July 1962): 144.

8 Charles Recolin, "The X-ray" in *The World Above the World*, ed. and trans. Brian Stableford (Black Coat Press Book, 2011), para 4, Kindle.

9 Ibid., para 26, Kindle.

10 Ibid., para 39, Kindle.

11 Edmond Hamilton, "The Man with X-Ray Eyes," *Wonder Stories* 5, no. 4 (November 1933), 388.

12 Ibid., 393.

13 *X: The Man with X-ray Eyes*, directed by Roger Corman (Metro-Goldwyn-Mayer, American International Pictures, 1963), 0:10:42 to 0:10:53.

14 Ibid., 0:04:00 to 0:04:07.

15 Ibid., 1:14:49 to 1:15:20.

16 Ibid., 1:15:42 to 1:15:46.

17 Ibid., 1:15:47 to 1:15:58.

18 Keith Phipps, "Roger Corman Reflects On His Long, Legendary Career–But He Isn't Finished Yet," *Uproxx* (May 5,

2017), accessed October 7, 2022, https://uproxx.com/movies/
interview-roger-corman/.

19 Kelsey Belle, review of X-Ray Camera–X Ray Vision Scan,
October 11, 2020.

20 fluffywolf SILLYcake, review of X-ray Scan Filter Cam, March
13, 2022.

Chapter 4

1 Nick Veasey, *Inside Out* (Stockholm: Bokförlaget Max Ström,
2017), 2.

2 Alan Burroughs, *Art Criticism from a Laboratory* (Little Brown
& Co., 1938), 56.

3 Ibid., 84, fn 18.

4 Ibid., 52.

5 Suzanne Muchnic, "Exorcising the Ghost of Art," *Los Angeles
Times* (June 25, 1995): https://www.latimes.com/archives/la
-xpm-1995-06-25-ca-17044-story.html.

6 "Marilyn Monroe's Chest X-ray Offered at Auction," *The
Telegraph* (April 12, 2010): https://www.telegraph.co.uk/news/
celebritynews/7582112/Marilyn-Monroes-chest-x-ray-offered
-at-auction.html.

7 Donald J. Trump @realdonaldtrump, "Those Tweets were NOT
Racist. I don't have a Racist bone in my body!" July 16, 2019,
8:59 a.m. tweet, https://twitter.com/realDonaldTrump/status
/1151129281134768128.

8   Morgan Gstalter, "Ex-senator challenges Trump to get
    X-rays proving he had bone spurs during Vietnam draft,"
    The Hill (March 21, 2019): https://thehill.com/homenews/
    administration/435212-ex-senator-challenges-trump-to-get-x
    -rays-proving-he-had-bone-spurs/.

9   Report "Hitler as Seen by His Doctors" (Vol. 2), 29 November
    1945, 57320060R, World War 2, 1939–1949, National Library
    of Medicine, Bethesda. https://digirepo.nlm.nih.gov/ext/dw
    /57320060RX2/PDF/57320060RX2.pdf.

Chapter 5

1   Chevalier Jackson Collection, *Mütter Museum*, accessed June
    25, 2022, https://muttermuseum.org/exhibitions/chevalier
    -jackson-collection.

2   Mary Cappello, *Swallow: Foreign Bodies, Their Ingestion,
    Inspiration, and The Curious Doctor Who Extracted Them*
    (New York: The New Press, 2012), 104.

3   "Food Irradiation: What You Need to Know," *U.S. Food &
    Drug Administration*, February 17, 2022, accessed July 12,
    2022, https://www.fda.gov/food/buy-store-serve-safe-food/
    food-irradiation-what-you-need-know.

4   Ibid.

5   Munchies Staff, "Stop X-raying Your Kid's Halloween
    Candy," *Vice*, October 29, 2015, accessed July 7, 2022, https://
    www.vice.com/en/article/jpad94/stop-x-raying-your-kids
    -halloween-candy.

6   Joel Best, "Halloween Sadism," *Joel Best*, accessed July 7, 2022,
    https://www.joelbest.net/halloween-sadism

7   Liz Mullen and Mary Gilstrap, "Hospitals Offer to X-ray Treats for Halloween," *Los Angeles Times*, Oct 30, 1985, accessed July 7, 2022, https://www.latimes.com/archives/la-xpm-1985-10-30-vw-12200-story.html.

8   Ibid.

9   Brendan I. Koerner, *The Skies Belong to Us: Love and Terror in the Golden Age of Hijacking* (New York: Broadway Books, 2013), 46.

10   Ibid., 47.

11   Yoav Gonen, "NYPD has super-secret X-ray vans," *New York Post*, Oct 13, 2015, accessed July 12, 2022, https://nypost.com/2015/10/13/nypd-has-secret-x-ray-vans/.

12   CPSC Case Number 181068767, Treatment Date October 10, 2018, *National Electronic Injury Surveillance System*, accessed June 28, 2022.

13   Ibid.

14   CPSC Case Number 210905066, Treatment Date April 12, 2021, *National Electronic Injury Surveillance System*, accessed June 28, 2022.

15   CPSC Case Number 210759723, Treatment Date July 17, 2021, *National Electronic Injury Surveillance System*, accessed June 28, 2022.

16   *Seinfeld*, season 6, episode 21, "Fusilli Jerry," directed by Andy Ackerman, written by Larry David, Jerry Seinfeld, and Marjorie Gross, featuring Jerry Seinfeld, Julia Louis-Dreyfuss, Michael Kramer, Jason Alexander, and Jerry Stiller, aired April 27, 1995.

17   CPSC Case Number 211220405, Treatment Date December 2, 2021, *National Electronic Injury Surveillance System*, accessed June 28, 2022.

INDEX

Blackface

An Essential Non-Fiction Book of 2021, *New Statesman*

12 Best Non-Fiction Books About Black Identity and History, *Book Riot*

Book of the Week, *Times Higher Education*

2022 Prose Awards Finalist, Media and Cultural Studies Category

> A truly eye-opening, defiant, must-read."
>
> — *West Emind Best Friend*

> Wide-ranging and hard-hitting . . . a passionate, well-informed, and gripping read . . . another triumph for Object Lessons."
>
> — *New York Journal of Books*

> Examines Hollywood's painful, enduring ties to racist performances."
>
> — *Variety*

> Sharp . . . in explicitly laying out the history and costs of blackface performance, [Ayanna Thompson] fully meets her stated aim of offering an accessible book that constitutes part of an ongoing 'arc toward justice.'"
>
> — *Times Higher Education*

Burger

Burger draws on an accessible combination of history and pop culture to reconsider America's obsession with the molded-ground-beef sandwich . . . [It] explore[s] alternative modes of offering cultural critique, pushing against traditional divisions between academic and popular writing, and between history and critique, in search of new, more palatable forms of packaging the unsettling stories behind the Anglo-American diet."

—*Humanimalia*

Burger is a work of advocacy as well as literature and cultural analysis."

—*New Orleans Review*

Best known for her groundbreaking *The Sexual Politics of Meat*, Adams would seem the least likely person to write about hamburgers with her philosophically lurid antipathy to carnivory. But if the point is to deconstruct this iconic all-American meal, then she is the woman for the job."

—*Times Higher Education*

Burger is a small book with a big punch . . . Adams approaches her topic as an animal rights advocate as well as a feminist . . . In this way, taking into account the lives of cows, as well as women, Adams convincingly explores the 'violence at the heart of the hamburger.'"

—*NPR: 13.7 Cosmos and Culture*

It's tempting to say that *Burger* is a literary meal that fills the reader's need, but that's the essence of Adams' quick, concise, rich exploration of the role this meat (or meatless) patty has played in our lives."

—*PopMatters*

Based on meticulous, and comprehensive, research, Adams has packed a stunning, gripping exposé into these few pages—one that may make you rethink your relationship with this food. Five stars."

—*San Francisco Book Review*

Doll

jaw dropping."

—*Is This Mutton?*

[Hart's] observations about how dolls are emotional vectors—simultaneously objects of scorn and adoration—are revelatory and relatable."

—*Brevity*

a fascinating personal and public exploration of the deeper meanings behind the plastic, polymer, and porcelain playthings that still shape American girlhood."

—Susan Shapiro, New York Times bestselling author of *Unhooked, Five Men Who Broke My Heart*, and *Barbie: Sixty Years of Inspiration*

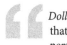 *Doll* is a heartfelt, intimate, and clever study of objects that terrify some and thrill others . . . giving us new perspective on these tiny, fragile mirrors."

—Allison Horrocks, co-host of the *Dolls of Our Lives* (formerly titled *American Girls Podcast*)

High Heel

Best Fifteen Books of March 2019, *Refinery29*

Best Nonfiction Books of 2019, *Paste Magazine*

 [B]risk, readable . . . Brennan circles around the shoes from all angles, and her brief chapters add up to a kaleidoscopic view of feminine public existence, both wide-ranging and thoughtful."

—*Jezebel*

 High Heel is poetry in prose, and while a serious work about the shoe in worldwide history and contemporary culture, it sounds more rhythmic, like poetry in motion."

—*San Francisco Book Review*

a properly modern consideration of what is at stake and it uses thoroughly intriguing methods of inquiry to approach a well-balanced lack of resolution."

—*PopMatters*

From Cinderella's glass slippers to Carrie Bradshaw's Manolo Blahniks, Summer Brennan deftly analyzes one of the world's most provocative and sexualized fashion accessories in *High Heel*... Told in 150 vignettes that alternately entertain and educate, disturb and depress, the book ruminates on the ways in which society fetishizes, celebrates, and demonizes the high heel as well as the people, primarily women, who wear them . . . Whether you see high heels as empowering or a submission to patriarchal gender roles (or land somewhere in between), you'll likely never look at a pair the same way again after reading *High Heel*."

—*Longreads*

High Heel is thought-provoking meditation on what it means to move through the world as a woman. Brennan's book, written in very small sections, is short, but powerful enough to completely change your world view."

—*Refinery29*

Hood

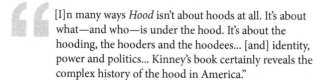

[I]n many ways *Hood* isn't about hoods at all. It's about what—and who—is under the hood. It's about the hooding, the hooders and the hoodees... [and] identity, power and politics... Kinney's book certainly reveals the complex history of the hood in America."

—*London Review of Books*

From executioners in modern-day Florida, to the Ku Klux Klan, to 'hug a hoodie' Cameron—this scholarly study explores a complicated cultural history . . . [Kinney's] argument about the connection between hoods and power is a strong one . . . The book is at its best on the connections between hoods and marginalized communities."

—*The Guardian*

[S]hort but ambitious... This provocative [book]... raises more questions than it seeks to answer—but that's fitting when the issues it discusses are still so urgent and so open."

—*Times Literary Supplement*

> In spry and intelligent prose, Alison Kinney tours the many uses of the hood in human culture, exploring seemingly unconnected byways and guiding the reader through some surprising connections. The ubiquitous hood, she shows, is an artifact of human relationships with power, the state, and one another. By the end of my time with *Hood*, I had laughed out loud, sighed in exasperation, and felt by turns both furious and proud."

—Rebecca Onion, *Slate Magazine*

Hyphen

> The hyphen . . . has inspired not one great book but two: *Meet Mr. Hyphen (And Put Him in His Place*, a classic by Edward N. Teall, published in 1937, and *Hyphen*, by Pardis Mahdavi, which came out in 2021."

—Mary Norris, *The New Yorker*

> Mahdavi's compelling histories offer guidance for a way out of a struggle that binds us all within so many unhelpful and frankly boring binaries. The book rules."

—*The Stranger*

Sewer

Get ready to dive into the wondrous underworld of waste . . . It's perfect for the fatberg fan in your life."

—*Mental Floss*

Hester goes deep on a topic that few relish[—]the inner workings of wastewater infrastructure—all to answer questions of how human habits are reshaping the environment, and what needs to change.

—*Bloomberg CityLab*

Takes readers on a journey underground to the meandering pipes and waterways underneath us where waste ferments and disease percolates. The oft-forgotten and hidden-but-so-necessary infrastructure below us has deep implications for urbanization, public health, infrastructure, ecology, and sustainability, not to mention our future."

—*Architect's Newspaper*

Souvenir

Souvenir, a sweet new book by Rolf Potts, is a little gem (easily tucked into a jacket pocket) filled with big insights . . . *Souvenir* explores our passions for such possessions and why we are compelled to transport items from one spot to another."

—*Forbes*

Souvenir offers ideas about what may be in play when we seek mementos . . . In the end, *Souvenir* suggests that the meaning of a keepsake is not fixed (its importance to the owner can change over time) and that its significance is bound up in the traveler's identity."

—*The New York Times*

Readers of this little treatise will never look at souvenirs the same way again. Five stars."

—*San Francisco Book Review*

A treasure trove of . . . fascinating deep dives into the history of travel keepsakes . . . [T]he book, as do souvenirs themselves, speaks to the broader issues of time, memory, adventure, and nostalgia."

—*The Boston Globe*

Sticker

Hoke . . . offers up an evocative reflection on queerness, race, and his hometown of Charlottesville, VA, in this conceptual 'memoir in 20 stickers.'"

—*Publishers Weekly*

Hoke's book uses stickers to chronicle everything from queer identity to the recent history of Charlottesville, Virginia—all of which should make this a book that sticks with you long after you've read it. (Pun intended, oh yes.)"

—*Volume 1 Brooklyn*

> Hoke's keenly constructed memoir-in-essays is really a memoir-in-stickers, from the glow-in-the-dark stars and coveted Lisa Frank unicorns of childhood to a Pixies decal from his teenage years."
>
> —*Electric Lit*

> *Sticker* is a trove of Millennial nostalgia. Its uniqueness lies not only in Hoke's unabashed storytelling but also in its critical analysis of American current events and its brutal honesty about a city rooted in racism . . . Hoke's writing is blunt and honest, and *Sticker* is a collection worth keeping."
>
> —Nicole Yurcaba, *Southern Review of Books*

Stroller

The Best Books of 2022, *New Yorker*

> For Morgan, strollers aren't just tools we use, or products we buy; they're dense symbols, with no single or settled meaning, of our relationships to parenting."
>
> —*The New Yorker*

Veil

Slim but formidable."

—*London Review of Books*

Rafia Zakaria, journalist and author, unravels the complex nexus of attitudes, policies, and histories revolving around this object in her fascinating new book, *Veil*. She demonstrates how the object can serve as a moral delineator, a disciplinary measure, a signifier of goodness, or as a means to subvert or rebel social norms. Through personal narratives and detailed analysis of various social and political conditions Zakaria offers an engaging and nuanced assessment of the veil in the contemporary context."

—*New Books Network*

I admired Rafia Zakaria's *Veil* months even before I read it . . . Her engaging prose is just what I hoped to find inside this little book, which is composed of short vignettes on the veil rather than a sustained philosophical treaty."

—*Reading Religion*